Yoga Sutras

The Means to Liberation

Translation and Commentary
by
Dennis Hill

Cover Design/Artwork by: Kathy Rottier

Order this book online at www.trafford.com
or email orders@trafford.com

Most Trafford titles are also available at major online book retailers.

Printed in the United States of America.

ISBN: 978-1-4251-4764-8 (sc)
ISBN: 978-1-4251-5982-5 (hc)
ISBN: 978-1-4669-5703-9 (e)

Trafford rev. 12/26/2014

Trafford PUBLISHING® www.trafford.com
North America & international
toll-free: 1 888 232 4444 (USA & Canada)
fax: 812 355 4082

Introduction to the Yoga Sutras

The Yoga Sutras were compiled about 2,000 years ago by the sage Patanjali from an oral tradition reaching back into unknowable antiquity. He gives us the essential wisdom for the practice of yoga and meditation to know, first hand, the essence of our true Self—the conscious indweller that enlivens this body. Experiencing the fully conscious state shows us the essential transcendent nature of the universe to bring us a state of undisturbed joyous tranquillity. Traditionally, this wisdom has been handed down from master to student as a transmission of the means to liberation.

The term "yoga" appeared in the Vedas long before Patanjali lived, but the Yoga Sutras stand in history as the first comprehensive treatise on the method of yoga and liberation. Patanjali speaks primarily from a point of view of the Samkya philosophy and the meditative Raja Yoga, giving us much of the Sanskrit vocabulary we see in the sutras.

Patanjali tells us that the pure blissful inner Self is already attained and all that is required is to lose interest in that which is not the Self. This is pretty straight forward, and we learn all we need to know in the first three sutras. Presuming we will not get it the first time, he goes on to detail the nature of the Self, the practices that will awaken us, the attainments that arise from the practices and then explains about the state of final liberation.

The first book begins by telling us that yoga is restraining the mind to a state of equanimity so that the mind is not disturbed as it surveys the appearance, and to know things just as they are. This teaching might be new information to today's yoga student who has come to understand yoga as fitness exercise. But Patanjali persists and explains the nature of the mind, the distractions in the mind, and the state of *samadhi* that arises when the yogi loses interest in the distractions.

Because of the enticements of the world the mind cultivates cravings for the pleasure, and aversion to the suffering brought on by the craving. Given the predominance of these influences, the mind just naturally does not rest in stillness. Book II on *sadhana* gives us practices to simultaneously draw out the inner bliss and quiet the distractions in the mind. In a concise practice of the 8 limbs of yoga, Patanjali packages for us the concept of *astanga*.

For the student who persists in the practices over a long period of time, various attainments, or yogic powers may arise. Patanjali describes these *siddhis* in some detail in Book III, but he says that we should not be distracted as we might lose our way on the path to liberation. It is best to just notice and continue on with *sadhana*.

Throughout the book we are reminded of two fundamental practices that lead to the final state, *kaivalya*. One practice is *vairagya* (dispassion, non-attachment) and the other is *viveka* (discrimination). In life, everything comes to us and everything leaves us. In both pleasure and pain we can welcome whatever comes, and release whatever leaves us. In the practice of *vairagya* we not only let go completely when it is time, but we do not become attached in the first place to whatever comes to us in the river of abundance. In the practice of *viveka*, we learn to discriminate between the mind and the watcher of the mind (consciousness itself). When we can rest in the state of awareness knowing itself, we know our true identity. Book IV (*Kaivalya*) is the story of the final outcome of these practices and insights as the yogi merges irrevocably into the bliss of the Self.

Dennis Hill

DEDICATION

I dedicate this work to THIS;
beyond which there isn't, without which we aren't,
and within which the self-luminous Absolute
appears as the diversity.
This work is dedicated to the Guru,
who teaches us
through silence, service, grace and reverence
that our very being is the supracausal divine presence.
This work is dedicated to true love, serenity and delight,
that spontaneously emerges
when one is steady in the inner contentment.

Book 1: Samadhi

1.1: atha yogā 'nuśāsanaṃ

Now, Yoga.

1.2: yogaś chitta vṛitti nirodhaḥ.

Yoga is the restraint of objectification by the mind.

This is one of the fundamental sutra of the entire work, so we will define these Sanskrit terms to better understand the aphorism and be prepared for usage of these terms in later references.

- *Yoga* can be defined as a discipline leading to identity (union) with the conscious Absolute.
- *Chitta* is an aggregate term that includes:
    - *Buddhi* - the intellect
    - *Manas* - instinctual imperative of acquisitiveness (de sires)
    - *Ahamkara* - the ego sense of individuality or separate ness

  This collective of psyche is also called the *Antahkarana.*
- *Vritti* is a mental process of objectification that mediates consciousness to its known objects; essentially a contraction of pure consciousness to imagine a word or visualize a form.
- *Nirodhah* is restraint or stilling.

The idea is simple; when the mind is restrained to equanimity (*sattva*), the unmoving seer becomes the predominant knower of the mind and the appearance. Once the mind is entrained to contentment by practice of meditation, the transcendent state gradually persists in our normal awareness in all circumstances. The mind is not different than the thoughts it thinks. Thus; no thought, no mind.

Here we see that Yoga has two facets: activity and state. The activity of Yoga is in restraining the mind to equilibrium, and the state of Yoga is that of the undisturbed seer.

1.3: tadā draṣṭuḥ svarūpe 'vasthānaṁ

Then the impartial witness abides in its own nature.

Once the mind has become purified through practice of meditation, the mind will not rush to interpret or dramatize the appearance; the customary inner chatter gives way to pure illumination of just what is. The impartial witness is the only one here to observe the outer or inner landscape. This is a very peaceful and happy state.

1.4: vṛtti sārūpyam itaratra

At times when restraint is not present, the Self identifies with the contents of the mind.

There are two identities of the Self: 1. The primary identity is the self-luminous impartial witness—the conscious indweller. 2. The contracted secondary identity is with *Antahkarana*.... The Self forgets itself and becomes distracted by *vrittis* arising in the mind. *Buddhi* cognizes name and form, *Ahamkara* arises creating a separate ego identity, and *Manas* instinctively reaches out to become involved in the imaginary drama.

1.5: vṛttayaḥ pañcatayyaḥ kliṣṭa akliṣṭāh

There are five kinds of vrittis that either cause mental affliction or lead to samadhi:

1.6: pramāna viparyaya vilkapa nidrā smṛtayaḥ

They are right knowledge (pramana), wrong knowledge, imagination, sleep and memory.

1.7: pratyakṣā 'numānā "gamāḥ pramāṇāni

Valid knowledge is direct perception (pratyaksha), verifiable deduction (anumana) and the word of one who has already reached the goal (agama).

The purest knowing is being conscious of Consciousness itslf—the Self knowing itself. Direct perception is, of course, seeing it with your own eyes. Verifiable deduction is a rational inference that can be proven in our own experience. The term *agama* generally means scriptural authority, but the words of a true guru is also considered *agama*.

1.8: viparyayo mithyā-jñānam atadrūpa pratiṣṭhaṁ

Wrong knowledge occurs when cognition is not in agreement with the substance of the reality.

We have all had the embarrassment of approaching someone we though was an acquaintance, to find a complete stranger. We just got it wrong. This is wrong knowledge. False knowledge is also caused by the five *kleshas* (afflictions): nescience, egoism, attachment, aversion, and fear of death.

1.9: śabda jñānā 'nupātī vastu-śūnyo vikalpaḥ

Thought that arises in the mind is imaginary.

To fantasize, "Roses are beautiful" is imaginary, as it is neither a direct perception nor is it a verifiable inference. To think, "This rose I hold in my hand is beautiful" is a direct perception, but is still *chitta vritti*: a thought construct in the mind. The word *water* does not quench the thirst; the thought of light does not dispel the darkness.

1.10: abhāva pratyayā 'laṁbanā vṛttir nidrā

Sleep occurs when psychic inertia is accompanied by cognition of nothingness.

The knowledge of the languid torpor of deep sleep is the mind knowing the void. The mind remembers whether sleep was fitful or serene. That is, sleep (*nidra*) leaves its impression on the mind.

1.11: anubhūta viṣayā 'saṁpramoṣaḥ smṛtiḥ

Recollection is the reappearance in the mind of a thing taken in before, and appears as a synthesis of the nature of the object and the process of knowing, producing the samskara.

The Sanskrit word "*klishta*" is the adjective form of the noun *klesha*, meaning trouble. Thus far in the Yoga Sutras, we understand that all *vrittis* are distractions from the state of Yoga. Now we see that some *vrittis* (*klishta*) are troublesome and others are relatively beneficial (*aklishta*). If *vrittis* take us away from Truth, then how is it that some *vrittis* are beneficial and can even lead us to enlightenment? Is this paradoxical?

All *vrittis* are the breeding ground of *samskaras* (latent impressions) that arise again and again, distracting awareness away from the bliss of the Self; directing subject to object. *Pramana* (valid knowledge) is *aklishta vritti* having a *sattvic* (peaceful) quality. The other types of *vrittis* have *rajasic* (active) or *tamasic* (inertia) quality, thus they are troublesome (*klishta*) *vrittis.*

Valid knowledge leading to awakening will be the last *vrittis* to go. Watch for the troublesome vrittis of imagination and memory; practice letting them go as they come up in the mind to minimize creation of latent impressions (*samskaras*). This will lead to a more *sattvic* meditation.

To summarize vrittis relative to their *Gunas* (attributes): **valid knowledge** is *sattvic*; **misunderstanding**, **imagination** and **memory** are *rajasic*; and **sleep** is *tamasic.*

I know there are numerous foreign terms here, but we will see them repeatedly throughout the Yoga Sutras. We can get familiar with them now, early in the book, so we can continue with good understanding. These terms will be most meaningful if you can relate them to experiences in your own meditation. For instance; categorize some of your thoughts according to the nomenclature given in Sutras 1.5 - 1.11. Or try to recognize the *Buddhi, ahamkara* or *manas* as they arise and stimulate trains of *vrittis* and *samskaras.* You will notice as you do this that you become somewhat detached to the emotional loading of the thoughts as you witness and analyze the arising and resorption of thought forms. Most important of all, though, is to experience your true self as the impartial witness. Practice this every day. Perfection is already attained, but mastery will come through the practice of Yoga.

1.12: abhyāsa vairāgyābhyāṁ tan nirodhaḥ

Chitta vrittis are restrained by practice (abhyasa) and non-attachment (vairagya).

In the path of Yoga, *sthiti* (steadiness of mind) is a very important concept. We attain *sthiti* through *abhyasa* (practice). A contemporary Siddha master said, "Meditation is to attain the steady state." From this vantage point we are undisturbed by the dramatic excesses of the world. We are utterly centered in equipoise. This centeredness is obviously the very opposite of tyranny by *chitta vrittis*.

1.13: tatra sthitau yatno 'bhyāsaḥ

Of these two, effort toward steadiness of mind is practice.

Patanjali begins the Yoga Sutras by saying that the state of Yoga is attained by restraining the mind to equilibrium. Now he tells us how: devoted practice and detachment. Very simple... there are only two things to do; meditate every day and cultivate selfless dispassion.

1.14: sa tu dīrgha kāla nairantarya satkārā "sevito dṛḍhabhūmiḥ

Practice becomes firmly grounded when well attended to for a long time, without break and with deep devotion (satkara).

In this sutra, *satkara* is translated as devotion. While this is good, there is more. In *satkara*, *sat* means Truth (existence as it is), and *kara* comes from the same root as *karma* (action). This gives us a word that means an action that reveals the truth of the Self, that pure light of consciousness by which everything is known. The purest devotion is toward knowing our Self as the divine inner presence. We can see our discipline of daily meditation as a heartfelt devotion rather than an obligatory task. Perhaps in the beginning meditation didn't fit our schedule, or we just didn't have time every day, or it was boring. Now we can be devoted to our practice. Examine how you really feel about it. We may be devoted to many things: our spouse, children, parents, even our dog. Include meditation in this good company; do this for yourself. Practice becomes firmly grounded when well attended to for a long time, without break and with *satkara*—deep devotion. Remember this: *Abhyasa* (the practice) is for a long time, without interruption, with your whole heart.

1.15: dṛṣṭa 'nuśavika viṣaya nitṛṣṇasya vaśīkāra saṁjñā vairāgyaṁ

When the mind loses all desire for objects seen or heard about, it acquires a state of utter desirelessness which is called dispassion.

Why do we need this practice of non-attachment? What is the cause of craving that disturbs the mind so much that Patanjali needs to give us this teaching? Since infancy we are conditioned to seek nourishment and satisfaction from outside ourselves. This conditioning (*samskara*) has persisted through our whole life. But now we are discovering that our own inner Self is the source of peace and happiness, though we have sought satisfaction through possessions, relationships, power, pleasure, love, influence, adventure, etc. All this is reaching out to the world to get something from it. We go through a life of many experiences and find that there is nothing out there that brings us enduring happiness.... Everything changes. When we look inward and discover that **pure awareness of just being** is filled with joyous tranquility, we have found enduring happiness that is there no matter what else is going on in the world. Merging into this peace and bliss requires daily practice to overcome our innate tendency to reach outward for satisfaction or pleasure.

1.16: tat paraṁ puruṣakhyaāter guṇa vaitṛṣṇuyaṃ

Knowing the innermost Self brings supreme non-attachment.

Ultimately we don't have to do anything to attain *vairagya* (dispassion; detachment) but hold to our meditative practice to reveal the source of all we ever thought we desired. Then there is nothing else to crave; we have found enduring happiness that is there no matter what else appears before us. In the fullness of the heart there is nothing else to desire. In this dispassionate state we enjoy whatever comes to us, and freely release whatever leaves us while attending to *dharma* in the world.

1.17: vitarka vicārā "nandā 'smitā 'nugamāt saṁprajñātaḥ

Samprajñāta samadhi—subject distinguishing object—is a progressive contemplation of reasoning (vitarka), concentration (vichara), joyful contentment (ananda) and awareness of just being (asmita).

The contemporary scholar Swami Hariharananda makes this observation: "*The successful concentration which brings knowledge cutting at the root of all afflictions is called samprajñāta-yoga.*" *Samprajñāta samadhi* is a crucial concept at this point in the Yoga Sutras, as it sets the stage for the next thirty three sutras. This is the base camp preparing us for the final ascent to the peak of the highest transcendent states of meditation. *Samprajñāta samadhi* is progressive because the meditator must pass through each stage of contemplation sequentially, beginning with *vitarka*.

Vitarka derives from the Sanskrit root *tarka*, which means vagrant thought, and is not really reasoning at all, but random undirected thoughts arising spontaneously in the mind. We have all seen these vagrants creep into our quiet meditation. *Kutarka* means negative thought, and is associated with reasoning in a negative vein. *Vitarka*, however, means *sattvic* thought related to truth in a peaceful context. So Patanjali is saying that the beginning of meditation is to be able to restrain our thought processes to positive and peaceful content. Once we can do this we can move on to concentration (*vichara*).

Vichara is a reflection or enquiry that comes in two flavors: *nirvichara* and *savichara*. *Nirvichara* is detached reflection on *tanmatras* (fundamental states of being) without attention to their qualities. *Savichara* is reflection with attention to quality. The most basic of the *tanmatras* are "I" and "that." In this sutra Patanjali implies *savichara*; reflection on the qualities of subject and object. The progression from *vitarka* to *vichara* is moving from *sattvic* contemplation of physical world objects, to focus on inner abstraction, such as the mantra.

Ananda is objectification of the inner feeling of sweetness that arises through practice of meditation, the mind being at peace.

Asmita arises when the mind is still, and one is simply aware of being the serene impartial witness—a naked sense of self-existence.

In this entire progression of meditative states, all are characterized by the process of objectification, the subject reflecting upon some object. Vagrant and *sattvic* thoughts are objects, bliss is observed as a feeling, even no-thought is perceived as this pure "I" having no thought. Subtle.

Generally, in *samprajñāta samadhi*, there is a current of energy flowing from subject (*Purusha*) to object (*Prakriti*), eternal to ephemeral; it is the impartial witness falling into partiality. This current of interestedness is the last impediment to transcendence.

Practically speaking we practice this progression of refined states in our own meditation, beginning with the concerted study of yoga philosophy (*vitarka*), the practice of the mantra (*savichara*), experiencing inner peace (*ananda*) and glimpsing the elusive inner stillness (*asmita*).

1.18: virāma pratyāya 'bhyāsa pūrvaḥ saṁskāra śeṣo 'nyaḥ

Asamprajnata samadhi is cessation of mentation (nirvikalpa) attained by supreme detachment (para-vairagya) leaving only latent impressions (samskaras).

Through the discipline of meditation practice, we progress through increasingly subtle objects of focus. *Asamprajnata samadhi* is the subject void of object. This is a radical leap from contemplating some object, to a thought-free awareness: consciousness, conscious of itself, shining.

Let us look more closely at the Sanskrit term "*nirvikalpa*." The root "*kalpa*" means passage of time, or a day of Brahman, which is a little more than eight trillion years. *Vikalpa* is thus "change over time." *Nirvikalpa* means literally "no change over time;" however, in common usage it usually translates as "thought-free meditation." Applying the transliteration to common usage we see that the experience of *nirvikalpa* will be that of unchanging stillness free of pertubation from *chitta vritti* or *samskara*. This is an important point because this sutra says that in *asamprajnata samadhi*, *samskaras* remain.

There are two levels to *asamprajnata samadhi*: the first is that the yogin will pass in and out of states of *nirvikalpa* where latent impressions will arise unbidden. After a long period of practice of *para-vairagya*, *samskaras* are as burnt seeds, never bearing fruit in the mind again. This is the second stage of *asamprajnata samadhi* also called *kaivalya*: liberation.

Para-vairagya is a practice of indifference to arising thoughts, while absorbed in the unchanging self-luminescence of pure awareness. Over time, *vrittis*, due to lack of interest, simply no longer arise leaving natural, persistent inner stillness. This is something we can apply to our own daily meditation: losing interest in whatever disturbs the stillness. This is difficult if we are interested enough in a thought to become involved with it, thus falling back into duality. We have to inspect our interest in arising thoughts and let go of our interest in them. Here we come to true detachment. Letting go of outer attachment is just practice for the real thing. Liberation is attained by the supreme detachment to interest in the inner flotsam and jetsam. This is not a practice to leave for later.

1.19: bhava pratyayo videha prakṛtilayānāṁ

Even awakened ones who have some mastery over mutable nature (Prakriti) return to take another body because of latent impressions.

As we continue our practice of meditation, our mastery increases over more and more subtle objects of contemplation. We build momentum of inner stillness, and absorption in our formless nature (*Purusha*). Through this momentum the *samskaras* lose potency and ultimately dissipate, never to return. If we leave the body before this final attainment, subtle attachments call us back to the objects of our interest. Once *vrittis* and fruit of latent impressions no longer arise, we are finished. We have attained liberation (*kaivalya*) from the wheel of karma to merge into the bliss of universal consciousness. If this state is attained while still in the body, we may not notice when the body falls away.

1.20: śhraddhā vīrya smṛti samādhi prajñā pūrvaka itaraṣāṁ

The path to asamprajnata samadhi is through śraddhā (trust), virya (vitality), smriti (remembrance), samadhi (concentration), and prajnapurvaka (discernment).

Śraddhā is commonly translated as "faith." However, because of the ambiguity of faith as belief in unverifiable concepts, we will think of *śraddhã* as trust. In this context, *śraddhã* implies a reverential trust in *agama* — the word of one who has already reached the goal. This includes both Vedic scripture and finished yoga masters. The student has reverent trust in *agama* because the teachings are verifiable in the student's experience.

Some scholars translate *śraddhã* as faith in the guru. We should understand just who the guru really is. A living master tells us: "The guru is not the *jiva* (body); the guru is *Shiva* (pure consciousness). The guru is not the *vyapti* (logical mind); the guru is the *Shakti* (power of consciousness to know itself)." Thus, we are directed to faith in our own inner presence of the Self.

Also; Yogacharya Hariharananda writes that *śraddhã* is certitude and true knowledge accompanied by tranquility. We will see *śraddhã* again in the Yoga Sutras, so contemplate these three views and synthesize your own comprehension about the meaning of *śraddhã.*

Virya is vitality; enthusiasm for *sadhana*; unbending intent to become established in the Self. Is the study of meditation, for you, an interesting concept; or a thrilling awakening to your true nature? Do you have *virya*?

Smriti is remembering to choose the impartial witness that is our essential nature over the duality of I/that. When we view the appearance with detachment, compassion and contentment we see the world as it is; we know the truth. *Smriti-sadhana* is cultivating the thought-free state (*nirvikalpa samadhi*) and remembering it as often as possible out in the world. *Smriti* is also an inner remembering of the veracity of these teachings. Do they seem somehow familiar? Do you just know that this is true? This is *smriti.*

Samadhi is a concentrated absorption in the object of meditation (*samprajnata*); or objectless meditation (*asamprajnata*).

Prajnapurvaka, a state of no determinate knowledge, is where the purest essence of the light of awareness is discerned. Also called discriminative enlightenment.

1.21: tīvra saṁvegānām āsannaḥ

The intent yogi may overcome obstacles rapidly.

The final state of bliss already exists within everyone all the time, thus it is possible that one may dispense with the veils of illusion and come to know the Self in a short period of time. If the yogi advanced to a late stage of sadhana in a previous incarnation, that *vasana* of attainment may be ready to resume, and complete in this lifetime.

1.22: mrdu madhyā 'dhimātratvāt tato 'pi viśeṣaḥ

The chances of success vary according to the degree of effort.

It must seem self-evident that the degree of self-effort is proportional to the result; this is our common experience. In earlier sutras we have explored exactly what that self-effort consists of and we know whether or not we have been diligent in these practices. But now there is a new word in the mix.... Surrender.

1.23: īśvara praṇidānād vā

Success is also attained by those who surrender to Isvara.

What method can be used to surrender to the sweet equanimity of the divine absolute? It works exactly the same as surrendering to sleep: be perfectly still and it will absorb you into itself. Perfect stillness of the body takes practice. Perfect stillness of the mind takes dedication. So what is it that is surrendered? It is the sense of separate identity: the ego. When the ego dissipates due to lack of interest, the impartial witness accrues no *karma* and is untroubled by the mind. This is liberation; to some degree or other.

1.24: kleśa karma vipākā 'śayair aparāmṛṣṭaḥ puruṣa viśeṣa īśvaraḥ

Isvara is supreme consciousness (Purusha), and is untouched by the afflictions of life, action and its result.

It is both frustrating and comical that the mind wants to know that which knows it; wants to define this mysterious divine conscious presence with words. Consciousness can know the mind but the mind can never know consciousness. Purusha, the Self, is the subject; the mind is merely an object of the seer. As we will see later, the mind (Buddhi) will learn to emulate the sublime serenity of the Self, but can only become it through surrender.

1.25: tatra niratiśayaṁ sarvajña bījaṁ

The intelligence of consciousness is boundless.

The Sanskrit root of the term "***Tatra***" is "***Tat.***" Tat means Consciousness Absolute. We see this word in the *mahavakya* "*Tat-tvam-asi*" in the Upanishads; which translates to "That thou art." We understand by this aphorism that our true identity is boundless pure consciousness, or omniscience. Typically we don't think of ourselves as omniscient, because it is the mind that is thinking this. The mind is not omniscient, but consciousness that is the observer of the mind, is. When the mind is still, and pure consciousness is at the forefront of observation, omniscience is present. Omniscience doesn't necessarily mean that we can recite the taxonomy of paleopiscetology or encompass the collected works of all scholars. Omniscience means being so clear that inspiration shines the light of Truth at every moment and we somehow just know the right action that is perfect in each circumstance. When the mind is undistracted by its own dream then we are totally open to the wisdom of divine omniscience. Our inner knowing is far beyond, and much greater than, the deductive processes and emotional knee jerks of the mind. The key is the clarity of the thought-free state (*nirvikalpa*).

1.26: sa pūrveṣām api guruḥ kālenā 'navacchedāt

The True Guru, Purusha, unconditioned by time, is the teacher even of the ancients.

We already know from the commentary on Sutra 20 who the True Guru is.... The guru is not the *jiva* (body); the guru is *Shiva* (pure consciousness). The guru is not the *vyapti* (logical mind); the guru is the *Shakti* (power of consciousness to know itself). The living masters teach us on the authority of their teachers, but ultimately, Yoga masters rely on their own experience as verification of the oral tradition handed down through a lineage that may go back thousands of years. These truths are verifiable and utterly unchanging.

Patanjali tells us here that *Purusha* is unconditioned by time, that is, not bound in some time dimension. How can this be? Isn't time pervasive in all existence? We can check the veracity of the time concept in the stillness of meditation. While the mind is quiet, notice if there appears any evidence at all of time: a linear progression of an event horizon flowing forward. You may find that "time" is a mere concept with no inherent existence. We experience persistence of being, but there is no passage of time in the timeless eternal now; the observer just is. It is only the mind that has dreamed up the inference that if a clock hand goes around, time must be real. It is a useful convention to be sure, but belongs to the ephemeral realm of change.

Purusha, our fundamental inner Self, is the primordial guru. In the stillness we know the timeless eternity of the unborn witness observing the world of change.

1.27: tasya vācakaḥ praṇavaḥ

The word designating the Self is the Pranava OM

The innermost blissful Self that we seek in the practice of meditation is, of course, nameless and formless. But we feel compelled to give it a name so the mind would have a way of recognizing its existence. Thus we have OM or AUM. It's pretty basic: open your mouth, vocalize, and you get "ah." Close it and you get "mmm." The "ooo" in the middle gives it character. Once the vocalization is finished, there is silence afterward. According to Vedanta philosophy it is this silence that is the real representation of the inner Self; it **is** the inner Self.

It should not pass without notice that in the search for a name for the divine *Purusha*, *satchidananda* is the only word that describes the experience of immersion in the inner Self. *Sat*: pure experience of just being. *Chit*: sentiency, consciousness aware of itself. *Ananda*: the blissful fullness of the thought-free state.

1.28: taj japas tad artha bhāvanaṁ

Repeat Pranava OM and immerse yourself in its meaning.

OM is called the *Pranava*; from the Sanskrit root *Prana*, meaning vitality, or that conscious energy flow that enlivens the body. The recommended method of practicing *Pranava* OM as a sacred mantra is to repeat the first two sounds (ah..oh) in passing, going almost immediately to sustain the mmm sound, then close it off and pause in the stillness. Repeat this silently on the in-breath and the out-breath for meditation. This practice not only displaces other thoughts in the mind but actually evokes the presence of the Self. What you feel in this presence is your true original nature.

The practice of constant repetition of the *Pranava* OM is called *mantra japa*. When it is set to music in chant it is called *swadhyaya*. We see here that Patanjali is giving us yet another practice for our *sadhana*. The first practice, given in Sutra 2, is restraint of *vrittis* in the mind, or meditation. The second practice (Sutra 12) is *vairagya*; non-attachment. Now we have *mantra japa* to sustain our focus on the divine *Purusha*.

1.29: tataḥ pratyak cetanā 'dhigamo 'py anatarāyā 'bhāvaś ca

From turning inward to the inner Self, obstacles are overcome.

Now we have the fundamental repertoire of practices to overcome the obstacles of distraction and will, in time, attain full awareness of our blissful nature. Patanjali does not say our life will be easy or that life in the world will go the way we want. The outer world is driven by *karma* and intention, but now there is certainty in our *sadhana* that we will succeed in the pursuit of inner peace and transcendence if we sustain our discipline of meditation, non-attachment and *mantra japa*.

1.30: vyādhi styāna saṁśaya pramādā 'lasyā 'virati bhrānti darśanā 'labdha bhūmikatvā 'navasthitatvāni citta vikṣepās te 'ntarāyāḥ

Distractions of the mind that are the obstacles to sattva and devotion are disease, dullness, doubt, carelessness, laziness, craving for pleasure, ignorance, failure in spiritual attainment, and slipping from a yogic state.

Patanjali lists nine *tamasic* (inertial) distractions that take us away from the *sattvic* state of Self-awareness. It is self-evident in our experience that each of these distractions occupy the mind to the exclusion of absorption in the equanimity of the impartial witness.

1.31: duḥka daurmanasyā 'ngam ejayatva śvāsa praśvāsā vikṣepa saha bhuvaḥ

Distress, despair, restlessness of the body, and disturbance of the breath arise and coexist with these distractions.

As if the distractions were not enough there are even worse conditions that arise as a result. Haven't these things happened to each of us at some point in life? Maybe even now? It's tough to meditate in the midst of all the turmoil. What to do?

1.32: tat pratisedhārtham ekatattvā 'bhyāsaḥ

Concentration on a single technique is the best practice to prevent or overcome the obstacles and their accompaniments

All the above obstacles to transcendence have one thing in common: the mind set that "I am this body." Patanjali gives us a practice in Sutra 1.23 that wipes away all distraction —*Ishvara pranidhāna* (Self-absorption in the supreme *Purusha*). The Self is never sick, dull, doubtful, careless, lazy, wanton, ignorant, or stuck; never distressed, depressed or disturbed. As long as we think we are the body, we are subject to affliction. Once we know our true nature as the conscious indweller that enlivens the body, we are suddenly free of all distraction... if we practice this devotion to our true nature, and become wholly the Self. It is not enough just to **think** we are the Self. We must surrender utterly; **become** the impartial witness every moment, in everything we do.

Patanjali does not specify in this sutra any particular practice; only that if you bear down on some practice he has given so far (meditation, *mantra japa, swadhyaya, pranidhāna*) the student will transcend the limitations of the mind and body to emerge fully in the divine Presence. This works.

1.33: maitrī karuṇā mudito 'peksāṇām sukha duḥkha puṇyā 'punyā viṣayāṇam bhāvanātaś citta prasādanaṃ

The mind becomes pure and calm by cultivating friendliness toward the happy, compassion for the unhappy, delight toward the virtuous, and benevolent indifference toward the unrighteous.

This sutra is eminently practical for maintaining the steady state while living in the world. Naturally we must actually practice this as a discipline so that we can observe the benefit of a pervasive peaceful state while dealing with the infinite variety of people we come in contact with. We may think it would be easy to befriend the happy, delight in the virtuous, have compassion toward the unhappy and indifference toward the unrighteous; if they were strangers or distant acquaintances. But what if the unhappy or unrighteous were in our own family living in the same house; or in the workplace? Could we maintain our composure of inner steadiness beyond the familiar drama with someone we have known a long time; practice compassion and benevolent indifference toward unhappiness and unrighteousness persisting right in front of us? Consider even the same person whose moods may vary among all these qualities... can we find the right key to maintain undisturbed calm through the changes?

Consider also the case of those whom we might have a mutual dislike. If they are happy, can we be friendly? If they are virtuous, do we take delight? Think about this. Do the practice and see what it feels like. Patanjali tells us it will be wonderful, and it will bring us to a sublime serenity.

It is likely that our inner peace will be tested most frequently by the unhappy. What does it feel like to maintain our personal steadiness being touched by other's negativity or anger? What inner feelings do we reach for in compassion? Can we find **detached sympathetic kindness**? Detachment insulates our serenity from entanglement with other's emotional drama. Sympathy affirms our heart's tenderness; and kindness will find a way to help the unfortunate in their time of discontent.

Now; what do we do about our own unhappiness? Just remember that it is only the ego that suffers; the Self is in bliss all the time. Chant the mantra, meditate, immerse yourself into the inner stillness that is the source of boundless joy and contentment. The impartial witness to our suffering is infinitely compassionate.

How much do we really want inner peace? Work with this self-evident practice in the most difficult situations and gain mastery of the steady state. We have come to meditation to awaken the deep inner serenity that lives always just behind the mind. We begin the quest in the safety of our personal meditation space; but ultimately we must take our discovery out into the world. In this sutra, Patanjali asks us to take our attainment into the light of day.

1.34: pracchardana vidhāraṅābhyāṁ vā prāṇasya

The mind is calmed by the controlled exhaling and retention of the breath.

Here we see for the first time in the Yoga Sutras reference to *prānāyāma*: regulation of the breath. There are many kinds of *prānāyāma* for different purposes. In the context of Yoga, it must be related to stillness of the mind. Remember from Sutra 2—the state of Yoga is no-mind.

Note that Patanjali references exhalation and retention, but not inhalation. The focus of the practice of *prānāyāma* (in the context of inner stillness) is control of the outbreath and allowing the inbreath to fill naturally with no effort at control. Remember that yogic breathing is abdominal, not in the chest.

Here is a basic *prānāyāma* practice to still the mind: In this practice, the *mantra OM* (or *Om Namah Shivaya*) is expressed silently on the outbreath, but not on the inbreath. Begin with a comfortably full inbreath, then exhale slowly and evenly to the natural end of the breath, not forcing residual air. The control here is concentration on evenness of exhalation, while the *mantra* floats above the breath. When the mind is focused on the quality of evenness, the mind will naturally be at rest and the *mantra* will occupy the mental space.

Evenness can be enhanced by slightly constricting the pharynx during exhalation so that easy control is gained over the rate of outbreath. Controlling the breath in this way brings a deeper focus of attention and stillness of mind. Patanjali goes into greater detail on *pranayama* in Book 2 (Sadhana) starting with Sutra 50. There he refers to the inbreath as *bahya*, the outbreath as *abhyantara*, and retention as *stambha*.

Now we come to the retention part. Retention is not a forceful holding, but just a pause at the bottom of the breath cycle to experience the stillpoint past the end of the *mantra*. Here we capture the perfect stillness and breathe it into our being during the natural filling of the inbreath. Again we reach the comfortable fullness and repeat the cycle of beginning the *mantra*, focus on evenness of exhale, end the *mantra*, pause in the stillness, then inhale the stillness back to the top.

This practice takes substantial concentration, but you will experience a more profound inner stillness than you would with *mantra* alone. Depending on your experience of it, you may want to continue this *prāṇāyāma* practice for the duration of your meditation. Or you may want to begin the meditation period with *prāṇāyāma*, then finish with *mantra-japa* or *nirvikalpa*, the thought-free state.

Finally, the controlled exhalation and retention should be integrated into a single process so that evenness is a feature of the entire breath cycle; thus preserving evenness of the mental presence.

1.35: viṣayavatī vā pravṛttir utpannā manasaḥ sthiti nibandhanī

Concentration on subtle sense perceptions can bring steadiness of mind.

Besides pranayama, there are other subtle yogic practices that can turn the attention inward, away from somatic, sensory or mental disturbance or obstacles. Such might be absorption in mantra or concentration on the light of consciousness itself.

To orient to this set of sutras please review Sutra 1.17 (*samprajnata samadhi*) that describes the progression of objective meditation from the gross to the most subtle. We see this progression reflected here: sense perceptions, inner light, detached state, finally the void of deep sleep. All these practices lead to steadiness of mind by complete absorption in the various objects over a significant period of time.

1.36: viśokā vā jyotiṣmatī

Or by concentrating on the supreme, ever-blissful Light within.

One can become absorbed in an inner lightness that is blissful and free from sorrow. An outcome of concerted focus to manifest a sensory phenomena is affirmation of progress along the way. We all need a sign that we are progressing, and breakthroughs may not come frequently. The phenomena is not the goal, but a means to mastery. As we gain mastery in ever more subtle concentrations we will ultimately have the skill to hold the steady state in a non-objective meditation as the impartial witness knowing just the Self.

1.37: vīta rāga viṣayaṁ vā cittaṁ

Or by concentrating with a mind free from attachment to sense objects.

Go deep and sense your purest heart; that aspect of yourSelf that is beyond disturbance. Concentrating there will ultimately take you to that place. In the beginning it may be helpful to meditate upon the mind of a great being who has transcended the obstacles to inner peace.

1.38: svapna nidrā jñānā 'laṁbanaṁ vā

Or by concentrating on a dream object or deep sleep experience.

If you should have an auspicious dream, concentrate on the revealed wisdom. Or even remember the deep peace of dreamless sleep.

1.39: yathā 'bhimata dhyānād vā

Or by meditating on anything one chooses that is elevating.

Over the course of sadhana we learn many techniques of centering and meditation. Choose any one that is simple and effective. As Patanjali said previously, focus on any one will dispel the distractions and return the meditator to inner serenity.

1.40: paramā 'nu parama mahattvānto 'sya vaśīkāraḥ

Gradually, one's mastery in concentration extends from something indivisible to the boundaryless infinite.

In previous sutras Patanjali tells us that concentration on elevating perceptions will bring steadiness of mind; thus we attain the power to bring the mind to stillness contemplating objects vast or small, ethereal or dense, still or moving. With this power, there is nothing that can disturb our meditation; everything is just as it is, being observed by the impartial witness. This is a rare and great attainment. Even so, it is not the attainment that is so great, it is the state of loving serenity that endures through all our experiences of living in the world.

1.41: kṣīṇa vṛtter abhijātasye 'va maṇer grahītṛ grahaṇa grāhyeṣu tatsthatad añjanatā samāpattiḥ

Just as a pure crystal assumes the color of a nearby object, so the mind with diminished vrittis becomes steady such that the knower becomes the known. This culmination of meditation is samadhi.

A mind absorbed in a liberated soul takes on the nature of that soul. A mind absorbed in the mantra is colored by the vibration of the mantra. Likewise, a mind absorbed in the knower of the mind reflects the quality of the knower. When the knower becomes the known, the mind (process of objectification) fades away leaving only transcendent consciousness knowing itself. This is *samadhi.*

1.42: tatra śabdā 'rtha jñāna vikalpaiḥ saṁkīrṇā savitarkā samāpattiḥ

Contemplation in which the knowledge of a thing is mixed with its name and meaning is called savitarka.

Early in the Yoga Sutras we are told that yoga is the restraining of thoughts in the mind. Well, precisely what is meant by *savitarka* as it relates to thought? Let's take this example: Consciousness, that sees through our eyes, becomes aware of a cup. This is knowledge (*jnana*). The mind (*antahkarana*) processes this knowing (see Sutra 1.2). The intellect (*Buddhi*) gives it a name "cup." Memory (*manas*) recalls, "This is not my cup, it belongs to Satya." The ego (*ahamkara*) says, "But I'm going to drink out of it anyway, because Satya is not here." Taken together, this process is *savitarka* — contemplation with thought. Looking at the constituents, we can discriminate the real from the imaginary. Real, true knowledge is consciousness aware of the cup (see Sutras 1.5 - 1.6). At the point that *antahkarana* becomes involved in processing the perception, *jnana* fades and illusion predominates in awareness as the ego follows the train of thought (*savitarka*). Then, either another train of thought arises, or awareness returns to *jnana*, true knowledge.

1.43: smrti pariśuddhau svarūpa śunye 'vā 'rthamātra nirbhāsā nirvitarkā

When the memory is purified, the object of concentration shines alone devoid of name and form. This is nirvitarka samadhi.

Purification of memory is the restraint of associative thought about the object of concentration. This restraint inhibits the ego from self-assertion, leaving only pure knowing of the object primary in awareness. Consciousness is undisturbed by the mind. The cup simply is what it is. To understand this practically, we can take the example of driving your car through town; but in a state of restrained thought. We observe the scene passing by, but we are not talking to ourself about it. We are simply paying attention to the traffic and the landscape undisturbed by chatter in the mind. This is *nirvitarka samadhi* driving the car. Reality appears, unlaundered by distortion. Otherwise we are like talking on the cell phone while trying to navigate a hazardous obstacle course.

1.44: etayai 'va savicārā nirvicārā ca sūkṣma viṣayā vyākhyātā

When the object of contemplation is subtle, samadhis of savichara and nirvichara can be distinguished in the same way.

Savichara samadhi is characterized by knowledge of a subtle object that is mixed with name and quality. *Nirvichara samadhi* is knowledge of a subtle object purified of attributes from the mind. Let us take the example of the mantra, as a subtle object. If we practice *mantra japa* while the mind is analyzing the meaning of the mantra, we have *savichara samadhi.* If *mantra japa* is practiced with thought-free awareness of the sound vibration only, this is *nirvichara samadhi.*

1.45: sūksma viṣayatvaṁ cā 'liṅga paryavasānaṁ

The most subtle objects of experience approach the indefinable.

Patanjali is taking us through a meditative progression from the tangible to the most subtle objects. It is easy to understand meditation on the tangible, but objectifying the subtler realms is more challenging. A thought (such as the mantra) is an object easily meditated upon. A state, such as bliss, is not too hard either, once the state has been experienced. This sutra says that the most subtle object has no name or form, but is the unmanifest principle of *Prakriti*; an objective void but with no form or content.

There are two kinds of stuff in the universe: matter/energy, and conscious awareness. Each has its own first cause. The unmanifest first cause of matter/energy is called *Prakriti*, the manifesting principle. The first differentiation from the Universal is *ahamkara* (ego). From ego arises mind (*chittam*), and from mind, the senses (*tanmatras*). This is the subtle hierarchy leading to the most subtle unmanifest object of meditation.

The first cause of conscious awareness is called *Purusha*, the quiescent, unmanifest, pure consciousness. *Purusha* is considered to be the pure spirit that enlivens the body. As such, it is not an object that can be meditated upon, as consciousness is the subject that is the seer of objects. In the literature we often see *Purusha* and *Prakriti* used together referring to the sum total of the universe: spirit and matter. Since consciousness is self-aware, we get a glimpse of meditation that transcends objectification of *Prakriti.*

1.46: tā eva sabījaḥ samādhiḥ

The foregoing samadhis refer to objects, tangible and subtle, but is not yet the final goal.

There are two levels of meditation: superficial and deep. Superficial meditation is absorption on that which has been objectified by the mind, whether it be a tangible object or a subtle state. These objects live on in the mind as *samskaras* (predispositions from past impressions) that can draw our focus back into the differentiated I/That state. Deep meditation is characterized by the purification of the *nirvichara samadhi* (thought-free awareness). The practice of this state purifies the *samskaras* so they no longer arise to disturb identity with the Self, witness of the appearance.

1.47: nirvicara vaisaradye 'dhyatma prasadah

Self-luminous radiance emerges in the purity of nirvichara samadhi.

In Sutra 1.17 we defined *nirvichara* as the detached reflection on the fundamental state of being without attention to quality. This is a very pure awareness that reveals the pristine Self in its boundless radiance. Here we find the steady state of inner peace that we seek.

Nirvichara samadhi is not a state we hide away in our solitary meditation, but bring into the world to live our life in. For most of the things we do, we don't need the mind gossiping about it. The purity of inner stillness is a better friend and gives us direct knowledge of what is at hand. The steady state of *nirvichara* always knows the Truth.

1.48: rtambhara tatra prajna

The undistracted awareness of nirvichara samadhi is filled with truth.

We can know things in several ways. Commonly we figure things out in the mind to get knowledge, often using the senses for information. This is valid (see Sutra 1.7), but is inferential. We also learn from others. This is good too, if we can verify it in our own experience. Now we come to transcendent, or direct knowledge. One example is perceiving an object with no thought in the mind about its name, appearance or function. We just receive the totality of the object and know it. Another example is knowing through intuition; it just comes to us and is true. We have all had this experience. A third example could be reading in the Yoga Sutras, or Upanishads, and have an inner knowing of its veracity... like a memory of its familiarity. Has this happened to you? This transcendent truth has several Sanskrit names; among then, *ritambhara prajna*, *nirvikalpa pratyaksha*, and *nirvichara samadhi*. We will see these terms again.

1.49: sruta 'numana prajna 'bhyam anya visaya visesa 'rthatvat

Truth of direct knowing is different from deductive reasoning or inference.

These are not uncommon experiences, but now we know they are a special case. It is through meditation that we fine tune our ability to evoke this great state of truth. As we glimpse the inner stillness time and time again, a momentum grows that wells up in our being and we begin to see with new eyes. We are not so quick to analyze everything to death but can wait patiently for the essence of the appearance to emerge in the stillness. Our intention to do this is the best way to overcome the inertia of conditioned *samskaras*, and will bring the light of truth to every minute of the day. It is here that knowledge becomes wisdom.

1.50: tajjah samskaro 'nya samskara pratibahdhi

The impressions of this samadhi will come to predominate over samskaras of distraction.

We have learned that *mantra japa* quiets the thoughts in the mind. Similarly, *nirvichara samadhi* dissolves the *samskaras* so that distractions from mental and emotional conditioning no longer arise.

When the mind attains to stillness, *mantra japa* is no longer needed. Just so, even transcendent wisdom falls away leaving only utterly pure awareness of consciousness itself. There is nothing beyond this; we have reached the fundamental groundstate of life and spirit.

1.51: tasya 'pi nirodhe sarva nirodhan nirbijah samadhih

When the impressions of even spontaneous self-awareness are transcended, there remains only the serene and undisturbed state of all-knowing wisdom.

Why would we want to attain such an austerity of mind? One reason might be to have undisturbed peace. There would never be any distraction, as the latent tendencies (*samskaras*) are as burnt seeds (*nirbija*). Another reason might be liberation from the wheel of karma. No further craving attracts no further incarnation.

Book 2: Sadhana

2.1: tapaḥ svādhyāye 'śvara praṇidhānāni kriyā yogaḥ

Self-discipline, study and recitation of sacred texts, and absorption in the true inner Self, constitute the essentials of Yoga in action.

Beginning Book One of the Yoga Sutras we learn that the state of Yoga is that of the undisturbed seer. Now in Book Two we see that the practices that lead us to the state of inner equanimity begin with *tapas*, or self-discipline. No surprise here. *Tapas* is often thought of as burning, or that which generates heat or energy. In this sense, yogic *tapasya* is the practice of conserving energy to direct it to the goal of Yoga. *Tapas* also implies endurance of hardship to keep focus on the path to liberation. All this *tapasya* is to purify the mind and body so that the state of Yoga is entered into with resolute will. A great change comes about in redefining relationships with our previous habits, notions and perceptions. The body is purified of imbalance and the mind is purified of mental and emotional clutter, leaving us strong and pure to get through these changes.

The second observance (*niyama*) of Kriya Yoga is *swādhyāya*: study and recitation of sacred texts, including *mantra japa*. It is obvious that scholarship alone does not lead to the state of Yoga. Before the fundamentals of Yoga were written down, they were passed down the generations in an oral tradition of recitation of the carefully constructed *sutras*. The vibration of the Sanskrit mantras in the texts were part of the practices leading to transcendent states. Also prescribed was repetition of specific *mantras (mantra japa)*, to embody the qualities of that *mantra*; as we shall see in Book III.

The third essential is *pranidhāna*, absorption in the inner Self (*Purusha*, conscious awareness). As we are able to locate the inner stillness and assume the persona of the impartial witness, we become identified with the Great Self while the small self of the mind and body becomes the helper rather than the tyrant.

This absorption is begun in the discipline of meditation, and realized when we become established in the steady state of the impartial witness. It is still us looking out through these eyes, but now we know we are the Self; the serene silent witness of the appearance.

2.2: samādhi bhavānārthaḥ kleśa tanū karaṇārthaś ca

Practicing these essentials, we overcome the obstacles and attain samadhi.

Yoga *sadhana* is also known as the Path of Discrimination (*viveka*): discernment of the Self from the ego. It is through the power of *viveka* that the our fundamental mistaken identity is burned away. This erroneous identity with our thoughts, feelings, body and personal history is gradually diminished through *tapas, swādhyāya and pranidhāna*. In the same way, we gradually become stronger in the awareness that we are the divine presence. It is not that the ego goes away, but it becomes channeled into a positive, supportive and peaceful attitude.

The power of *sadhana* is in the practices given in this second book of Yoga Sutras. Through these practices samadhi is attained, beginning with the *niyamas* (observances) of self-discipline, study and *mantra japa*, and devotion to the Self.

2.3: avidyā 'smitā rāga dveṣā 'bhiniveśāḥ

Nescience (avidya), ego, attachment, antipathy, and dread of death are the five obstacles (kleshas).

Isn't this somehow familiar? Look back at Sutra 8 of Book One, and we see listed these five *kleshas* of misunderstanding (*viparyaya*). Now in Book Two, Patanjali will explain in detail, these *kleshas* that bring us so much suffering, so it will sink in. In Sutras 4 - 10 the *kleshas* (afflictions) will be characterized; then in Sutra 11, Patanjali gives the practice that dissolves all obstacles, brings serene contentment, and liberates us from the wheel of *karma*. Ahhh.

2.4: avidyā kṣetram uttareṣāṁ prasupta tanu vicchinno 'dārāṇaṁ

Avidya (not knowing the Self) is the origin of the other obstacles, whether they are dormant, weakened, interrupted or sustained.

At this point it is essential to have a good understanding of Patanjali's usage of the term *avidya*. It is from the Sanskrit root, *vidya*. *Vidya* has three different, but related meanings:

1. Knowledge – as in knowledge about the arts, sciences or humanities.
2. Meditation – as a means to liberation. For example: *Brahmavidya* is meditation upon an aspect of the inner Self (*Brahman, Purusha*), such as given in the **Upanishads**.
3. Wisdom – the direct perception of the Self (*nirvikalpa*).

In the Sanskrit grammatic system, a word preceded by the letter "a" shifts the meaning to the opposite of the root meaning. Thus *avidya* is the opposite, or absence of *vidya*. The usage in this Sutra refers to the absence of the knowledge of the Self; the absence of wisdom. Thus, not knowing the Self causes egoism: mistaken identity with thoughts, feelings, the body, and personal history. Likewise, *avidya* causes the obstacle of attachment. Attachment arises out of the sense of lack or emptiness. As well, ignorance of the Self is at the root of antipathy, not seeing the Self of all in each person. Dread of death arises when one is unaware of that inner state of pure consciousness that endures beyond the death of the mind and body.

Kleshas are ***dormant*** in the very young before acquiring language which will obscure the reality and will give rise to the imaginary ego.

Kleshas are ***weakened*** in the Yoga student who is devoted to overcoming the limitations of the ego.

Kleshas are ***interrupted*** in the Yoga student who has attained partial mastery, but occasionally slips into a subdued *samskara*.

Kleshas are ***sustained*** in those who are not inclined (yet) to control the tendencies that hide direct perception of the serene inner Self.

2.5: anityā 'śuci duḥkhā 'nātmasu nitya śuci sukhā 'tma khyātir avidyā

Avidya is taking the ephemeral as eternal, the impure as pure, the painful as pleasant, and the non-Self as the Self.

Patanjali considers the fundamental ignorance as mistaken self-identity; and from this, proceeds all other errors in perception and understanding. This occurs naturally in our cultural conditioning: to seek outwardly for our identity, mistake the ephemeral as eternal, and discover that attachment to pleasure inevitably leads to disappointment. These errors are mitigated by seeking inwardly to the pure awareness of being as our true nature; knowing our Self to be the impartial witness. Suddenly we have a new reference for the eternal, experience true purity, and choose blissful contentment over attachment and aversion.

This is all very nice to know, but how do we make the leap from *avidya* to *vidya* (identity with the Self)? It begins with glimpses of inner stillness in meditation. Once we can string these glimpses together and have a sense of the presence of the witness just behind the mind, we can take this presence with us in our daily activities as the watcher of our actions. This is the beginning of discrimination (*viveka*) and non-attachment (*vairagya*) from the ego-mind that embodies this pervasive ignorance. As the impartial witness becomes stronger in our awareness we now have choices in our thoughts and actions as well as clear insights in our mental processes so we can direct our lives toward inner peace and living harmony. Ultimately we will attain full identity with the serene Self that we have always been all along.

2.6: dṛg darśana-śaktyor ekātmatevā 'smitā

Pure consciousness is the power of seeing, but the ego is confused, thinking the body/mind (the instrument of seeing) is the seer.

Let's look at who is looking. From **Sutra 2** in the first book we know that the ego is the "I" sense, and *Buddhi* is the intellect that synthesizes knowledge of objects, thoughts and feelings. Thus *Buddhi* is the instrument of knowing. Because of this role as the knower, *Buddhi* is commonly thought of as the seer; but this is not so. Immersed in the inner stillness of meditation, the impartial witness observes the *Buddhi* apprehending and digesting objects, subtle and tangible. If this is the case, then *Buddhi* is an object of awareness, and not the subject. Here we discern the fundamental error of our identity. The ego would like to be top dog, but it is being watched by our true Self.

Look at your thumb. You know the thumb, but the thumb does not know you. Similarly, the Self knows the mind, but the mind can never know consciousness (*chaitanyam*); because consciousness is the subject, not an object.

Now, what can we do to correct this stupefying error of identity? Standing in the great Self, looking out from the impartial witness reasserts our true identity and conditions us to the truth of our being. Since the mind/ego is not different than the thoughts it thinks, the more time we spend in thought-free equipoise, the more we become our authentic Self. We have spent our life identified with the contents of awareness (thoughts, feelings and personal history); it is time to know ourselves as awareness itself.

2.7: sukhā 'nuśayī rāgaḥ

Pleasure is followed by attachment. *[And attachment is followed by the pain of separation.*

Whatever comes to you <u>will</u> leave you. Everything changes.]

2.8: duḥkhā 'nuśayī dveṣaḥ

Pain is followed by aversion. *[And aversion is followed by constant fear.]*

See if what Patanjali says here is consistent with your experience. Look at your attachments and determine if they follow a pattern of pleasure: mental, emotional, physical or spiritual. Is it hard to be impersonal about these attachments? Are they distractions to absorption in the bliss of inner stillness? Now, look at your aversions. Are they avoidance of pain: mental, emotional, physical or spiritual? Is it hard to be impersonal about these aversions? Are they distractions to absorption in the bliss of inner stillness?

It is not likely that we can give up our attachments all at once; so how do we practice this *sadhana* of *vairagya* (non-attachment)? Some attachments might bring us peace and others, not. What about reverence for saintly persons (*shraddha*), love of friends, affection for family, compassion for those less fortunate? These are *sattvic* (peaceful) attachments and support our *sadhana* along this wisdom path of yoga. Other attachments are *rajasic* or *tamasic* (agitative or restrictive). We can begin by releasing our bondage to these non-*sattvic* attachments.

Okay, just how do we go about letting go of these *kleshas* (afflictions)? If we fight and struggle with these magnetic distractions, they become tar babies; every time you strike they stick to you more tightly. If, instead, you draw inward to the sweet stillness of meditation, the tar baby falls away through lack of interest. This takes practice to actually lose interest in that which causes you pain; simultaneously turning within to relish the divine equanimity. We remember from earlier Sutras that keeping company with inner stillness causes the *samskaras* to dissipate. In the midst of distraction from our attachments, turn inward; take refuge in the *mantra*, settle into the sweetness of the Self.

Eventually all attachments will need to be released to find peaceful contentment, and liberation from this wheel of *karma*. Begin with the non-*sattvic kleshas* and the rest will fall away easily, in time.

Really, you **can** love someone without attachment.

2.9: svarasavāhī viduṣo 'pi tathā 'ruḍro 'bhiniveśaḥ

Flowing through life is the fear of death, the clinging to life, and it is dominant in all, even the learned.

We all know this resistance to annihilation. The writers of TV crime dramas know we will feel something when their character begs, "Please don't kill me, I'll do anything!" Even in meditation, the ego/mind struggles against the nothingness. Why is this?

Yoga philosophy holds that for uncounted lifetimes we have met death in fear, and this impression (*vasana*) is retained into this incarnation. Even if you don't believe in karma and reincarnation, we know our trepidation about the unknown. And death is the final unknown.

For whom, however, is death unknown? For the ego? Certainly. For the impartial witness? Perhaps not. Perhaps the impartial witness **is** that state of consciousness that survives the death of the body. It is the teaching of yoga that: "Meditation is the end of fear." This is true because in meditation we cultivate that transcendent state that is not local to the mind and does not die when the body falls away. Mastery in the state of yoga liberates one from the final fear of death.

2.10: te pratiprasava heyāḥ sūkṣmāḥ

The subtle kleshas (obstacles to happiness) are destroyed by the cessation of the mind.

Listed again are the five *kleshas*:

1. Ignorance and misunderstanding (*avidya*)
2. Egoism (*ahamkara*)
3. Attachment (*raga*)
4. Aversion, antipathy (*dvesha*)
5. Fear, dread of death (*abinavesha*)

These *kleshas* arise because of misidentification of the Self as our thoughts, feelings, personal history, and the body. These mistaken notions arising in the mind create a continuous stream of drama about an imaginary ego. Once we experience the presence of the silent witness we can step back into that identity and begin to release the appropriated ego and its dramas. As the stillness pervades our being, the mind becomes serene and content. The *kleshas* begin thinning out through lack of interest by the impartial witness. The obstacles gradually subside into dormancy. When the mind becomes utterly still, the subtle *kleshas* dissolve completely. We emerge as the serene, blissful, liberated Self.

2.11: dhyāna heyās tad vṛttayaḥ

Fully developed kleshas can be overcome by meditation.

Consciousness becomes the mind, contracted by the objects of awareness. In meditation we learn to discriminate between the contraction of consciousness, i.e. thoughts; and consciousness itself, the observer of the mind. It is through this conscious discrimination that **ignorance** is replaced by the truth of direct knowing; the **ego** fades in the light of the impartial witness, **attachment** falls away in the presence of the Self; **antipathy** is pushed aside by joyous contentment; and the **dread of death** does not arise in the eternal present of here and now.

As the observer of the thoughts we recognize the developing drama in the mind and can be undisturbed by the power (*shakti*) of awareness appearing in the form of thoughts, feelings and erroneous identity. This is a gradual process, but every day we make progress when we touch that stillness in meditation and carry it with us into the world.

2.12: kleśa mūlaḥ karmā 'śayo dṛṣṭā 'dṛṣṭā janma vedanīyaḥ

Actions rooted in the five kleshas (afflictions) bring karmic consequences in this, or future, incarnations.

The literature of Yoga Philosophy tells us, generally speaking, that the actions we take have karmic outcomes. If we take action based upon the *klesha* of antipathy (*dvesha*) then we reap what we sow. If, on the other hand, we perform an act of generosity based upon the *klesha* of egoism (*ahamkara*), this brings abundance. But how do we transcend karma altogether, empty out the well of karmas (*karmashayah*), and become liberated in this lifetime (*jivanmukta*)?

We are told that actions based upon right understanding (Sutras 1.6, 1.7) incur no karmic outcome. As well, meditation destroys the *samskaras* that give rise to the five *kleshas*. To list the essentials of right understanding:

1. direct knowing from the Self (*pramana*)
2. direct perception (*pratyaksha*)
3. verifiable inference (*anumana*)
4. the word of one who has already reached the goal (*agama*)

These principles translate to leading a life of virtue rooted in the practice of meditation. Really, this is available to us right now in this very life of work, family and yoga. The outcome is a cessation of suffering in the present, release from karmic debt in the future and an inner life of peaceful contentment.

Is there some general guideline by which we might measure our daily life, minute to minute, to see if we are on track? We can examine who is the doer of our actions. If we find ourselves doing whatever is needed without drama or burden, then the Self is the doer, and no karma or suffering will accrue. Drama and burden is our thumbnail litmus test of right living. Be the watcher of your mind as you go through the day and see why you do the things you do, and who is the doer of these actions.

2.13: sati mūle tad vipāko jāty āyur bhogāḥ

When the karmic root remains, its fruition is rebirth, span of life and experiences of pleasure and pain.

Samskaras (latent impressions of mental and physical actions) manifesting from some *klesha* (affliction), is called a *karmashaya*. If it is a virtuous *Samskara*, it results in a beneficial karma in this or another lifetime. If it is a harmful *samskara*, the resulting karma brings unhappiness now or later. These karmas can be cancelled by an opposite action, burned out by yoga *dharma*, or reinforced. If a certain *karmashaya* persists through more than one life, it is called a *vasana* and results in rebirth, a certain span of life, and related experiences of pleasure and pain.

We see that at every step along the way a *samskara* can propagate into suffering and rebirth, or it can be burnt out and never bear fruit again. A *samskara* present in a restrained mind will die from lack of interest. A *samskara* of right understanding never bears *karma*, as it generates pure action.

2.14: te hlāda paritāpa phalāḥ puṇyā 'puṇya hetutvāt

The karmas bear fruits of pleasure and pain caused by virtue and harm.

Generally speaking, karmas return to us because of our attachment to outcome of actions; be they virtuous or harmful. Actions rooted in ignorance, ego, attachment, aversion or fear find us again, in this incarnation or another. Selfish desires that bring us pleasure strengthen the *samskaras*, thus their *vasanas* persist through numerous lives until they are burned out through *sadhana*.

Remember also that actions performed in the state of the impartial witness are free from *karma*. Even immersed in the dream of the ego, pure actions taken with no attachment to outcome likewise bear no fruit.

2.15: pariṇāma tāpa saṁskāra duḥkhair guṇa vṛtti virodhāc ca duḥkham eva sarvaṁ vivekinaḥ

The discriminating person knows that attachment to worldly objects leads to fear, anxiety, reinforcement of samskaras and constant change.

Through attachment to the pleasure of possession of objects, wealth, and relationships, suffering is the inevitable outcome. With discrimination (*viveka*) we experience that all these things come to us naturally, but they also leave us in time. Looking for happiness in attachment to pleasure is the cause of suffering. We all know the anger of betrayal, the frustration of expectation and the grief of loss. Why do we persist in this suffering? Perhaps it's cultural; everyone does it. But you have stepped upon this path of yoga, the path less traveled by. There is hope of transcendence of the commonplace.

Renouncing objects, wealth and relationships does not end the suffering. All these things come and go as a natural part of life, but attachment is the *klesha* that corrupts everything that comes to us. True renunciation is simply letting go of attachment and giving ourselves fully to the *dharma* of whatever comes to us; then, ultimately, we easily release whatever leaves us.

In Sutra 7 of this book we began to detach from the *rajasic* and *tamasic kleshas* because they are easier than the *sattvic* afflictions to release. Now we are at the part where we release attachment to the *sattvic* afflictions (reverence, love, compassion).

Love is not something we do to someone else; love is something we are. In the depths of meditation we feel the sweetness of just being. This is the love of our nature. A great saint tells us: "**Love is motiveless tenderness of the heart**." If we are in this state of motiveless tenderness, aren't we loving everyone we touch? There is nothing else to do about it. It is the *dharma* of relationship to be centered in the heart, to be motiveless in action and tender in our affection. It's not a great leap to think we can be motiveless and tender, and at the same time be unattached to the outcome of our actions. This is a powerful and life-changing practice that begins with meditation and ends with happiness every moment and freedom from the *karmic* cycle.

What is the basic fear in relationship? That we will be abandoned? The bliss of the Self will never leave us. Who we truly are is perpetually happy and content.

2.16: heyaṁ duḥkham anagatam

The suffering that is yet to come may be avoided.

The pain that is referred to in this sutra is future *karma* generated by actions rooted in the five *kleshas* resulting in *vasanas* that perpetuate into future incarnations. According to Vedanta, there are three classifications of *karma*:

1. ***Sanchita karma***: The sum of all *karmas* of this life and past lives.
2. ***Parabdha karma:*** That portion of *sanchita karma* that is bearing fruit and shaping the events and conditions of the current life, including physical attributes, personal tendencies and associations.
3. ***Kriyamana karma:*** The *karma* being created and added to *sanchita* in this life by one's thoughts, words and actions.

Sanchita karma can be burned away by the grace (*diksha*) of a living master, and performing the prescribed *sadhana* of self-discipline, study and *mantra japa*, and absorption in the Self given in sutra one of *Sadhana Pada*. *Parabdha karma* that is unfolding now must be lived through. We may arrest the accumulation of *kriyamana karma* by non-attachment to outcome of action and by the *sadhana* of *tapas, swadhyaya* and *pranidhana.*

In short, if we meditate and know the Self, we burn out past *karmas* and live peacefully, free of suffering in the future. After all, it is only the ego that suffers; and even if painful karma accrues to us, if we are indifferent to it, where is the suffering?

2.17: draṣṭṛ dṛśyayoḥ saṁyogo heya hetuḥ

The cause of avoidable suffering is the illusion that the seer is the same as the seen.

In general, we tend to identify with the contents of awareness rather than awareness itself; that is, we are absorbed in our thoughts, feelings, personal history, and the body as our identity. These elements are part of nature like all other constituents of the physical universe (*prakriti*). Nature is constantly changing, so is the mind constantly changing. There is no stillness, no peace, until we recognize the impartial witness just behind the mind: the observer of the appearance.

There is purpose in the unsteadiness of the mind; it is seeking stillness and repose. It will not rest until it finds peace. Through meditation it overcomes the restlessness and enters into the bliss of sublime contentment. Let us have a new appreciation of the torture of the mind; ultimately attachment and fear brings us transcendence. The purpose of suffering is to create the longing for its opposite. Think about it. In your deepest hurt, don't you wish for some way out, some means to escape the suffering? We discover in meditation that it is only the ego that suffers, and we are not the ego; we are the transcendent Self that is in bliss all the time. In this way we extinguish the illusion that the seer is the same as the seen. We now know that the seer is the mute witness of the appearance. *Purusha*, the eternal subject, awakens to the time-bound mutability of *prakriti*. The suffering is forever finished.

2.18: prakāśa kriyā stiti śīlaṁ bhūte 'ndriyāmakaṁ bhogā 'pavargārthaṁ dṛśyaṁ

The experienced world consists of the elements and the senses in play. It is of the nature of cognition, activity and inertia, and is for the purpose of experience and realization.

Beginning the **Yoga Sutras** we learned of the subject (impartial witness: *Purusha*) and object (material world: *prakriti*). As well, we see in Chapter Thirteen of the Bhagavad Gita, Krishna teaching Arjuna of the ***the field*** and the ***knower of the field***. These concepts have been verified as real in our experience through the practice of meditation as well as common observation.

Now we will abstract these concepts to their constitutional principles. The next few sutras will explore these high level principles (*tattvas*) of yoga philosophy; beginning with *prakriti*. One thing we must keep in mind is that in reality, *Purusha* is the immutable unchanging and *prakriti* is the mutable changing. *Purusha* will be explored as the eternal knower of being, and *prakriti* will be shown as the ephemeral substance of nature that comes and goes in and out of existence, on many scales. It is considered that the eternal *Purusha* is the "real," and ephemeral *prakriti* is "not real" in its essence.

Prakriti consists of both the tangible world of nature (mediated by the senses) as well as the intangible objects of the mind, that is: thoughts and feelings. All objects of *prakriti* are inherently a mixture of qualities. These qualities are called by Patanjali, *prakasha* (light of illumination), *kriya* (activity), and *sthiti* (inertia). In contemporary parlance this cluster of qualities is also know as the *gunas: sattva, rajas* and *tamas*. For this discussion, however, we will stick to the original Sanskrit nomenclature.

In nature, observed by *Purusha*, the qualities are never found singularly. All objects have a mix of the qualities, although one typically predominates to give the object its characteristic nature.

Prakasha, here, means knowable by *Purusha*. This includes the tangible, intangible, subtle, unmanifest, even potential manifest and unmanifest. So everything in *prakriti* embodies the quality of knowableness. *Kriya* means all knowables that have an active nature. Similarly, *sthiti* objects are, by nature, at rest, inert.

All *prakriti's* objects and their qualities aggregate into the appearance for the entertainment of *Purusha*. The only problem is that the appearance, mitigated in the mind by *Buddhi*, is subject to nescience, ego, attachment, aversion and fear. Absorption in the drama of the ephemeral is the veil over the eternal witness of the appearance. It is when the witness (*Purusha*) loses interest in the changing *prakriti* and becomes self-aware that liberation is at hand. Thus the purpose of the manifestation of *prakriti* is to lead *Purusha* back to itself through the stinging pain of the *kleshas*. Turning within, the Self is revealed and *prakriti* is seen as simply the play of consciousness (*chitshakti vilas*). *Purusha* awakens from the long dream of the unreal.

When we dream, things appear solid and people appear real. What happens in the dream seems real, apparent pleasure and pain brings us joy or grief. When we awaken, we see that we have created an imaginary drama within our own consciousness and not any of it was truly real. In exactly the same way we shall awaken from the long-dream of this incarnation and realize that the vivid play upon the screen was merely a play of consciousness; whimsy of divine sport. The object of the game is to wake up before we die or our fascination with the mirage will bring us back to the dream to pick up where we left off.

2.19: viśeṣā 'viśeṣa liṅgamātrā 'liṅgāni guṇaparvāṇi

The three gunas -- prakasha, kriya and sthiti -- have four stages: the manifest (visesha), the subtle (avisesha), the primary (lingamatra), and the unmanifest (alingani).

We humans have a curious nature; we like to ask "why?" and "what is the cause?" This inquiry then evolves a related nomenclature of name and form (*nama-rupa*). This is true of science, humanities, philosophy, even mysticism. We know from the previous sutra that objects in the knowable universe have characteristic qualities. The current sutra is the tip of the iceberg of a vast nomenclature of objects and qualities, and their evolutionary hierarchy. Rather than expounding a scholarly lexicon of nomenclature, let us take an empirical approach to making these stages real for us, from the gross to the sublime.

Beginning meditation we sit quietly and are aware of the visible, audible, tactile and aromatic environment. This is the manifest stage of knowables, or *prakriti*, with all their qualities apparent (*visesha*).

Next we close our eyes and withdraw our reach of perception to the inner stillness. In this subtle stage, we are still aware, but the impressions are not the focus of our attention (*avisesha*). This is the stage of the pure I-sense; just the awareness of existence. This stage just below the manifest, we will call the subtle. Here, *prakasha* is the predominant guna, *kriya* and *sthiti* are recessive.

In the next deeper level of meditation, *prakriti* is neither existing nor non-existing, neither real nor unreal, consciousness is primal and uncontracted by any objects, subtle or manifest. *Prakriti* is latent, known by inference, but still knowable.

At the unmanifest level, *prakriti* is present but the *gunas* are in perfect equilibrium, thus not manifest. The meditator is aware only of awareness itself. There is no content to contract consciousness from its own bliss.

As you close your eyes for meditation, be aware of the stages passing before you as you descend into the depths of the Self.

2.20: draṣṭā dṛśimātraḥ śuddo 'pi pratyayā 'nupaśyaḥ

The indweller is pure consciousness only, which though pure, sees through the mind and is identified by ego as being only the mind.

Conscious intelligence is the eternal light of awareness by which everything else is known, and has the power to know itself. Consciousness itself is the life of sentiency; it is how we are alive. The mind is confused about this, however, and believes it is the seer. The mind (*antahkarana*) is comprised of *Buddhi* (intellect), *manas* (root of desires) and *ahamkara* (ego). Of these, *Buddhi*, the thinker, thinks it has awareness. But it is consciousness that becomes the *Buddhi*, contracted by the objects of perception. *Buddhi* is ephemeral *prakriti*, consciousness is eternal *Purusha. Buddhi* dies with the body, consciousness is untouched by death. More immediate than that, in the stillness of no thought, the mind goes utterly out of existence; the mind being no different than the thoughts it thinks. The *Buddhi* notices this and, being the discriminative faculty, realizes the truth that the mind is not the Self. Thus begins the awakening of the yogi to the path of liberation (*kaivalya*).

2.21: tad artha eva dṛśyasyā 'tmā

The very existence of the seen is for the sake of the seer.

In yoga philosophy the fundamental endowment of knowable creation is to be the object of *Purusha*. If this is so, then the existence of an object is dependent upon *Purusha*, the observer. Thus, if an object can not be observed, then it no longer manifests, but is not destroyed. Revelation of an object for observing is a function of the *Buddhi*. Experience is only a form of *Buddhi*. Remembering that *Purusha* becomes *Buddhi* contracted by an object of perception, we see how this works.

2.22: kṛtārthaṁ prati naṣṭaṁ spy anastam tad anya sādhāraṇatvāt

Although the seen is dead to him who has attained liberation, it is alive to others because it is common to all.

When we live as the impartial witness, the appearance of an object in perception does not automatically contract consciousness into activity of the mind, thus we are essentially dead to that object; as it is unmanifest to *Buddhi*. If this object awakens a *vasana* of the mind stimulating associated thoughts and memories, the liberated state fades and *Buddhi* once again becomes associated with *Purusha*.

In the clarity of deep meditation we can watch this little dance of the mind coming into and going out of existence with the emergence and resorption of thought objects. At some point in our *sadhana* the *vasanas* will thin out then disappear forever, leaving us permanently established in the liberated state (*kaivalya*).

2.23: sva svāmi śaktyoḥ svarūpopalabdhi hetuḥ saṁyogaḥ

Purusha—the experiencer—is identified with Prakriti—the object of experience—in order that the true nature of both Prakriti and Purusha may be known.

Let us look closely at the relationship of seer and seen. The association of *Purusha* and *Prakriti* produces cognition. The resulting knowledge is of two kinds; (1) experience of pleasure and pain, and (2) liberation. We see that both forms of awareness are states of alliance between *Purusha* and *Prakriti.* When liberation is attained, the two are separated. *Purusha* alone remains as the impartial witness to the appearance.

2.24: tasya hetur avidyā

This identification is caused by avidya (nescience).

In the liberated state both right and wrong knowledge cease. Wrong knowledge, *vasanas* of imbedded *kleshas*, no longer arise. Right knowledge, the discrimination of *Purusha* from *Buddhi*, also ceases because *Buddhi* no longer exists. *Kleshas* of nescience, ego, attachment, aversion and fear are destroyed by discriminative knowledge (*viveka*) and supreme detachment (*vairagya*). Even discriminative knowledge dissolves its own existence as fire consumes its fuel.

2.25: tad abhāvāt saṁyogā 'bhāvo hānaṁ tad dṛśeḥ kaivalyaṁ

Liberation (kaivalya) is the dis-association of the seer and the seen, that brings the disappearance of ignorance (avidya).

Purusha (seer) is not inherently bound to *Prakriti* (objects of awareness), it only seems that way because of conditioning of the immature psyche. In the practice of meditation we are able to restrain the *vrittis*, awaken to the inner stillness, and discriminate the silent Self from the chaos of vagrant prattle. Once we know the stillness and know we are the Self, we can detach our identity from contents of awareness. Ignorance fades and wisdom emerges. This brings the end of association of *Buddhi* with *Purusha*; this is liberation.

2.26: viveka khyātir aviplavā hano 'pāyaḥ

The persistent practice of discriminative knowledge is the means to liberation.

Discriminative knowledge means we are established in the identity of *Purusha*; we live from the perspective of the great Self. **Persistent** means we never forget. *Buddhi* never again spews chatter about the appearance; the emotional roller coaster has come to rest. The body is the temporary abode of the indweller as it runs out *karma*. Yet we live in the world, we are diligent in the *dharma* of our family, occupation and society, and we follow the *sadhana* of this yoga of wisdom.

What is it really like to live in the liberated state? Those who know, seldom speak of it. But we get a rare glimpse through the pen of the great sage Valmiki. In the six volumes of Valmiki's epic **Yoga Vasishta** (V:53), the sage Vasishta gives us something to look forward to if we are persistent in meditation:

> Purity, total fulfillment of all desires (hence, their absence), friendliness to all, truthfulness, wisdom, tranquility and blissfulness, sweetness of speech, supreme magnanimity, lustrousness, one-pointedness, realization of cosmic unity, fearlessness, absence of divided-consciousness, non perversity—these are my constant companions. Since at all times everything everywhere happens in every manner, in me there is no desire or aversion towards anything, whether pleasant or unpleasant. Since all delusion has come to an end, since the mind has ceased to be and all evil thoughts have vanished, I rest peacefully in my own self.

2.27: tasya saptadhā prānta bhūmiḥ prajñā

Steady wisdom manifests in seven stages.

The first four stages comprise freedom from action. The final three relate to liberation of the mind.

1. The beginning of the Yoga path is filled with learning and knowledge in the mind. This is good, but it reaches a point of diminishing returns. The last thing to learn is that to progress further, the mind must be still. Restraining the *vrittis* is the first stage and one that triggers a cascade of the next six stages. In other words, inner stillness is the gateway to any further attainment. However, once there, the final state will come in due course.

2. In the second stage, the obstacles to happiness (*kleshas*) have been largely dispersed, and there is no need to continue putting effort toward seeking or restraint.

3. Identity is completely shifted from the ego (*Prakriti*) to the Self (*Purusha*) and the yogi lives fully in direct knowing, not requiring rational constructs.

4. *Dharma* is transcended in this stage. Nothing further is prescribed to do, as the yogi is no longer the doer. Actions happen as appropriate and the ego no longer drives activity.

5. *Buddhi*, the cognitive aspect of the mind has fulfilled its purpose of reflecting the phenomenal world and discriminating Self from non-self.

6. With *Buddhi* dissolved, the mind is at rest. *Vasanas* are burnt away and, with contentment, there is no further craving for the world.

7. In the final stage *Purusha* is free of relationship with the *gunas* of *Prakriti*. The Self rests within itself, free and self-luminous.

We need not think of the attainment of steady wisdom as far off; after all, it is already attained. *Sadhana* is just the process of getting out of the way of our already fully realized nature. Just as in the beginning of meditation we were able to see glimpses of stillness, we also have glimpses of each of the seven stages given in this sutra. Over time these glimpses grow into their fullness, as we persist in *sadhana*.

2.28: yogāṅgāṅuṣṭhānād asuddhi kṣaye jñāna dīptirā viveka khyāteḥ

By the practice of the limbs of Yoga, the impurities are destroyed and there dawns the light of wisdom, leading to discriminative discernment.

In this introduction to the eight limbs of yoga, Patanjali refers to transcending the five obstacles to happiness: nescience (not knowing the Self), ego, attachment, aversion and fear. These obstacles (*kleshas*) are progressive, in that nescience (*avidya*) strengthens ego which becomes immersed in attachment, aversion and fear. Sutra 1.2 tells us that yoga is the restraint of thought in the mind. It is this restraint that awakens Self-knowledge and, in turn, diminishes the suffering of the ego brought on by attachment, aversion and fear. Patanjali suggests that by practicing the eight limbs of Yoga that the student will attain the wisdom of the Self and ultimately, discrimination of the silent witness (*Purusha*) from the noise of the world (*Prakriti*).

2.29: yama niyamā 'sana prāṇāyāma pratyāhāra dhāraṇā dhyāna samādhayo 'ṣṭāv aṅgāni

The eight limbs of Yoga are:

1. *Yama (restraints)*
2. *Niyama (observances)*
3. *Asana (posture)*
4. *Pranayama (regulation of breath)*
5. *Pratyahara (sense withdrawal)*
6. *Dharana (concentration)*
7. *Dhyana (meditation)*
8. *Samadhi (transcendent superconsciousness)*

The first four of these practices are external and the final four are internal. The natural starting points of Astanga Yoga are (1) *asana* that will stabilize, strengthen and purify the body, and (2) *dhyana* that will purify the mind. As the practice of *asana* progresses, all the other limbs of Astanga must be integrated as well. Simultaneous with *asana*, we must learn and follow the *yamas* and *niyamas* as well as sustain a daily discipline of meditation. If equal emphasis is placed on both the external and internal practices, Astanga Yoga will blossom into an integrated life of health and happiness.

As we progress through the study of the Yoga Sutras devoted to Astanga, each practice will be taken individually in different sutras, but we must not neglect the other practices in our personal development. *Asana* and meditation will be the foundation practices as we study the restraints and observances. Asana practice will integrate *pranayama*, and meditation will integrate *pratyahara*, *dharana* and *samadhi*.

Through this integrated approach, health and happiness will gradually emerge as our predominant state to carry us forward into purity and transcendence: the goal of yoga.

2.30: ahiṁsa satyā 'steya brahmacaryā 'parigrahā yamāḥ

Yama consists of non-violence, truthfulness, non-stealing, moderation, and non-covetousness.

What is the purpose of the *yamas* and *niyamas*? Is it to make us better citizens? What does it really matter whether I always tell the truth or not? The real effect of developing these virtues is that they bring us inner peace; it quickens the inner stillness. This is the core practice of yoga. If you intentionally harm someone, does it bring you peace? If you crave something that you do not have, does it bring you peace? What is your real experience about this? These practices are not just rules that someone else tells us to follow; these practices awaken the bliss of our true inner Self. You will see.

The individual restraints are explored in detail in Sutras 2.35-2.39.

2.31: jāti deśa kāla samayā 'navacchinnāḥ sārva bhaumā mahā vrataṁ

These Great Vows are universal, not limited by class, place, time or circumstances.

It is typical that these vows are taken by monastics in various orders of monks and are absolute. Patanjali was a monastic and we see here his utter commitment to the vows. At the time these sutras were recorded from even more ancient sources, they were intended for renunciate yogis. But what if we are a householder and have not taken monastic vows? It is only reasonable to assume some flexibility from the absolutes of these vows. We can examine ourselves to see what we want out of our study and practice of Astanga Yoga. For higher aspiration, a deeper commitment will be required to these *yamas*, *niyamas*, meditation and *asana* practices. You choose.

2.32: śauca saṁtoṣa tapaḥ svādhyāye śvara praṇidhānāni niyamāḥ

Niyama consists of purity (saucha), contentment (samtosha), self-discipline (tapas), study and mantra (swadhyaya), and absorption in the inner Self (Ishvarapranidhanam).

Purity in mind, word and action brings us into alignment with the Self, which is the beacon of purity.

Restraint of thought (*vrittis*) through meditation brings purity of mind. In the stillness we awaken to the inner joy that is always there just behind all the drama.

Purity in word is a great kindness; and it is not so difficult to be kind. Purity of action is having no expectations of outcome, and incurs no *karma*.

All things come to us in life; we can welcome whatever comes and release whatever leaves us. This brings great contentment without the drama of craving, attachment and aversion. Take notice of what disturbs your meditation. Isn't most of it just being malcontent; wanting things to be different? Contentment is wonderful; cultivate this.

In ancient times, *tapas* was associated with penance and endurance of hardship. Life was very hard then, often brutal. But now life is easier. Great self-discipline, however, is still required in the path of Yoga. The observance of *tapas* means persevering in our practices, bearing up as we go against the grain of our conditioning, and maintaining equipoise in the face of great change.

In meditation we are able to locate the inner stillness and assume the persona of the impartial witness. This is absorption in the inner Self.

2.33: vitarka bādhane pratipakṣa bhāvanaṁ

If thoughts arise that are contrary to the virtues of yama and niyama, the opposite state should be cultivated (pratipaksha bhavana).

The opposite of a negative or destructive state of mind is the state of yoga; that is, the state of *sattvic* mind. When the mind is beset by contrary thoughts the best recourse is to step back into the thought-free state (*nirvikalpa*) of sublime equanimity, the impartial witness of the mind. If the student is not yet at a stage of meditation where *nirvikalpa* comes easily, then we can take refuge in the *mantra*. *Mantra-japa* of the *Pranava*, OM; or the *maha-mantra* of yoga, *Om Namah Shivaya*, will soothe the savage ego and return it to the *sattvic* state. Thus the destructive thoughts will not manifest into harmful action, to yourself or others.

A practical benefit of daily discipline in meditation is that the state of Yoga is present, or at least fresh in memory so that if contrary thoughts should arise, their opposite (*pratipaksha bhavana*) is close at hand. Test this in your own experience.

2.34: vitarkā hiṁsādayaḥ kṛta kāritā 'numoditā lobha krodha moha pūrvāka mṛdu madhyā 'dhimātrā duḥkhā jñānā 'nanta phalā iti pratipakṣa bhāvanaṁ

Contrary thoughts and emotions such as those of violence—whether done, caused to be done, or even approved of—indeed, any thought originating in desire, anger or delusion, whether mild medium or intense—do all result in suffering. Neutralize such a state through its opposite.

Such destructive thoughts left untransformed by *pratipaksha bhavana* emerge as actions that will cause suffering, to yourself or others. If the impulse to action is felt, suffering can still be avoided by returning to the blissful contentment of the Self. Reach for the *mantra*, take a quiet moment to peer out through the eyes of the impartial witness. The drama of the mind will subside and you will remember the sweet inner presence of your true Self.

2.35: ahiṁsā pratiṣṭhāyāṁ tat saṁnidhau vaira tyāgaḥ

When one is established in harmlessness (ahimsa), those near are at peace.

The virtue of *ahimsa* is not attained through practice of nonviolence. This observance is born in meditation. When one becomes established in undisturbed inner peace then harmlessness is practiced effortlessly in the world. Not only is the yogi undisturbed by provocation but the state itself is a calming force that shines in one's company.

This principle is true of all the observances and restraints. The virtues arise in the state of the meditator and are then practiced in the world with no effort. We might say that the virtues of *yama* and *niyama* are built-in to the Self; that is its nature. All that happens in sadhana is that the conditioned mind gets out of the way to allow the true nature of the Self to emerge; the veil of ignorance (*avidya*) falls away. The only attainment is surrender to that which has always been our Self.

2.36: satya pratiṣṭhāyāṁ kriyā phalā śrayatvaṁ

When the yogi is firmly established in truth (satya), the power of fruitful action is acquired.

One grounded in truthfulness gains will-power and potency of thought and speech. Not only what one says is true, but what one says becomes true. It becomes so through no action. Even though willful, *satya* transcends *karma*.

2.37: asteya pratiṣṭhāyāṁ sarva ratno 'pasthānaṁ

When the yogi is firmly established in honesty (asteya), riches present themselves.

One feature of *asteya* (literally non-stealing) is impartiality. Knowing the Self through meditation we become the impartial witness. Thus one lives established in *asteya* effortlessly. Riches (*ratna*, literally, jewels) are of two kinds: inner riches and outer riches. An honest person naturally draws outer riches, as people are more inclined to share generously with one they trust. The inner wealth is simply the state of blissful contentment that is persistent through all experience of one established in the Self.

2.38: brahmacarya pratiṣṭhāyāṁ vīrya lābhaḥ

When one is established in moderation (brahmacharya), spiritual vitality (virya) is gained.

Let's look closely at the term *brahmacharya*. The Sanskrit roots are *char*, meaning "path," or "to move;" and *Brahman* meaning "the Absolute," or "Truth." Literally, *brahmacharya* means the path to Truth, or movement toward the Absolute. Here, "Truth" is defined as the light of consciousness by which everything else is known; and awareness knowing itself. Our experience of this in meditation is the power (*shakti*) to focus on awareness itself, beyond the contents of awareness.

In earlier times *brahmacharya* took on the meaning of sexual abstinence for the monastics. Later it became non-promiscuousness, as householders came to the path of Yoga. Today (except for monastics) it is commonly used in the context of moderation in all things, including sensuality, to enhance spiritual vitality.

We know in our own experience that extremes of anything disturb meditative stillness and our *sadhana*. It is also self-evident that moderation helps us focus on our path to living as the great Self, and gives us vitality for the practices.

With moderation in all things there will be less disturbance of the mind bringing us closer to restraint of thought as given in Sutra 1.2 *Yogas chitta vritti nirodhah.*

2.39: aparigraha sthairye janma kathamtā saṁbodhaḥ

When the yogi is confirmed in nonpossessiveness (aparigraha), there arises knowledge of the "how" and "why" of existence.

Meditation takes us to the conscious groundstate of our true being. From this perch of pure awareness we become detached from objects that make up the contents of awareness; objects like the body, conditioning in the mind and the story drama of ego. Looking out from this purity of stillness we know who we are, why we are here and what our purpose is for the future. We know this because consciousness is not constrained by space-time, and we are that transcendent consciousness.

Possessiveness points us outwardly to clutch onto the stuff of the world. When we release our grasp and just let the world be as it is, we can turn inward with total openness to the joyous tranquility of the Self. Confirmed in this state, through long practice, our sense of self is transformed from the imagined limitations of the ego to boundaryless illumination of the Self.

2.40: śaucāt svā 'ṅga jugupsā parair asaṁsargaḥ

From purity follows a withdrawal from enchantment over one's own body as well as a detachment from contact with others.

Living in this world we devote much energy to satisfaction of our desires, finding comfort and pleasures, and attainment of our goals. All this seeking is to find fulfillment in the outer physical plane. Coming to yoga turns us inward to the richness of a subtle plane of being. We begin finding satisfaction, comfort, even attainments that were previously hidden. This great adventure focuses on purifying ourselves of wrong understanding, deeply imbedded conditioning and attachments to the world.

Many practices for purification are given in the Yoga Sutras: *asana, pranayama, dhyana*. Purification happens on several levels: the physical body, pranic body, subtle body and causal body to reach awareness of the supra-causal. The net effect of this process of purification is that all the satisfaction we craved in the outer world is fulfilled in this inner path. Thus we naturally turn away from attachments to things and people to enjoy peace, contentment and joy of the Self. In this, we seek simplicity and solitude.

2.41: sattva śuddhi saumanasyai kāgrye 'ndriya jayā 'tma darśana yogyatvāni ca

From mental purity there arises cheerfulness, power of concentration, control of the senses, and a fitness for Self-realization.

We can characterize mental purity by contentment, mental stillness and joyous equanimity. In contentment we are happy with our sense of being; not necessarily dependent on outer circumstances for our well-being. In this cheerful contentment we are not distracted by the mind so are able to focus concentration in the direction that *dharma* takes us. Likewise the body is not distracted by craving pleasure, which we know is the precursor to disappointment or worse. Our focus in life graduates from approval in society to delight in the Self.

2.42: saṁtoṣād anuttamaḥ sukha lābhaḥ

Contentment brings supreme happiness.

To find happiness we must discriminate between inner and outer contentment. Since the outer world is the domain of change, contentment may not be desirable or even possible. It is best not to use this sutra as an excuse for complacency or avoidance of dharma.

The inner contentment **is** desirable and possible. But what are the causes of inner discontent? Only the mind is discontent, as the Self is ever content. In the mind that is entangled in desire for what is not, attachment and fear, there is no peace. To know the uninterrupted happiness of contentment of the Self, the mind must be restrained to equanimity through *asana* and meditation.

2.43: kāye 'ndriya siddhir aśuddhi kṣayāt tapasaḥ

Austerities (tapas) destroy impurities; and with the ensuing purification of the body and sense organs, physical and mental powers (siddhis) awaken.

In Sutra 2.1 we see that *tapas* is concentrated self-discipline in *sadhana* that arises from burning aspiration for liberation. This often requires endurance of hardship as the body returns to balance through *asana* and *pranayama*; the mind purifies of conditioning through meditation; and our whole being transmigrates to identity with the Self. Simple, yes. Easy? Not very!

But what is this about supernormal powers? This sounds pretty good. Looking ahead we see a whole section of sutras on how to develop yogic powers. While it is true that *siddhis* come through the process of purification and austerities, the purpose of this process is to become the embodiment of the blissful Self. If our purpose is to develop imperious powers, Sutra 3.51 tells us that taking pride in any of these accomplishments does not lead to the Self, but brings a return to nescience, ego, attachment, aversion and fear.

To take the natural course of wisdom we persevere in our self-discipline. As *siddhis* manifest, we notice; then return to *sadhana.*

2.44: svādhyāyād iṣṭa devatā saṁprayogaḥ

Swadhyaya is a direct means to absorption in the divine presence.

The Sanskrit term *swadhyaya* is a complex term that includes study of the philosophical literature, self-study, recitation of scriptural text, and personal *mantra japa*. This practice brings right understanding, immersion into Sanskrit phrases—the vibration of which acts to purify the subtle body, and evokes the deity of the *mantra*. The net effect of this cluster of practices turns one inward to the experience of the divine presence: blissful serenity of the conscious indweller. This should be practiced every day so there is continuity, momentum and an awakening of the great Self within represented by the deity of the *mantra*. *Swadhyaya* is a very powerful practice, and will bring transformation.

2.45: samādhi siddhir īśvara praṇidhānāt

Samadhi is attained through surrender (Ishvara pranidhana) to the Self.

Patanjali is persistent in this theme of ***Ishvara pranidhana*** (surrender, or immersion in the Self). Previously in sutras 1.32 and 2.32 we see that this is the direct path to the highest state of Yoga. What does this mean, exactly, to surrender? What do we do, and what state is this? Simply stated, it means for the ego to get out of the way of the silent witness—the conscious indweller. When we look out on the world it is the Self that is seeing and knowing. The ego, with its neediness and fear, has subsided. This is the state of *samadhi*; the culmination of the eight limbs of Yoga.

As a practical matter, how do we live in the world in *samadhi*, without the ego? We know we are surrendered to the Self when our predominant presence is inwardly quiet, and our actions are performed without burden or drama. This is not hard; it's just that we are not accustomed to being this way because of our social conditioning. After all, this really is our true nature. The practice of *Isvara pranidhana* simply awakens us and reconditions us to remember who we are. See for yourself; after a period of practice don't you seem to remember this state as familiar? Be patient with yourself. If you persist in the practices as a discipline, *samadhi* will arise in its fullness.

2.46: sthira sukham āsanaṁ

Asana should be a steady comfortable posture.

It is known that Patanjali did not practice or teach Hatha Yoga. Rather, he followed the meditation path of Raja Yoga, a Samkhya tradition. For him, *asana* was any posture (such as *Siddhasana*) in which one could sit for meditation that is steady and comfortable (*sthira-sukham*). It was not until 1,500 years later (~1,300 c.e.) that Yogi Svatmarama codified the hatha postures in his Hatha Yoga Pradipika, a *Tantric sadhana* (based upon Goraknath's Siddha Sidhanta Paddhati). In the Hatha Yoga Pradipika, *asanas* for purification of the body is paramount, and activation of *Kundalini Shakti* is fundamental. Neither of these practices are mentioned by Patanjali. So we see that the term *asana* is framed quite differently in the two traditions.

Astanga Yoga presented in the Yoga Sutras was popular in India for at least 300 years before Patanjali wrote his aphorisms describing this culture of pragmatic philosophy and practices. *Asana*, in *Astanga Yoga*, is a means to something far greater than physical culture alone. *Asana* is a pose for sustaining meditation. In the care of a competent instructor, each posture will become steady and comfortable so we may forget the body entirely as we enter *samadhi*.

The illumined state is infused with stillness; but the mind cannot become still until the body is still. In the practice of *asana*, the body, having attained stillness, teaches the mind the same stillness. Similarly, the mind can never become steady and comfortable until the body is so conditioned. Each *asana* is a meditation posture, and each meditation is an *asana* of the mind.

2.47: prayatna śaithilyā 'nanta samāpattibhyāṁ

Asanas are perfected by relaxation of effort and meditation on the Infinite.

On the 8-limb path, *asana* is the vehicle to transcendence. In the beginning, *asana* can be uncomfortable, even painful, depending upon the skill and experience of the student. But in time, one can relax into the pose, being grounded with spine erect, to redirect awareness inwardly. At this stage relaxation is effortless and steadiness is sustained naturally, bringing perfection to the *asana*.

Meditating on pure awareness of just being, the body sense dissolves into the void. We have the experience of transcendence being free of the limitations of space-time. When awareness is withdrawn from the body, spatial dimensions are no longer relevant. When the mind is still, there really is no evidence of the time dimension, but only awareness of persistence of the eternal present.

2.48: tato dvandvā 'nabhighātaḥ

When asasa is mastered there is a cessation of the disturbances caused by dualities (dvandva).

The duality (*dvandva*) that has been Patanjali's primary focus thus far in the sutras is pleasure/pain on one side of the coin, and bliss of the Self, on the other. But there are other dualities that are balanced in *asana* mastery and in restraint of the *vrittis*. We come to maintain indifference to heat and cold, praise and blame, loss and gain, hunger and satiety, *vidya* and *avidya* (knowledge and ignorance), *raga* and *dvesha* (attachment and aversion). When poise on the physical plane and one pointedness on the mental plane are attained, the pairs of opposites fall away as obstacles to transcendence.

Even though Hatha Yoga was developed much later than Patanjali's *Astanga* we find *Tantric* concepts that also fit this sutra. The opposites of *ida/pingala* (feminine/masculine), *apana/prana* (inbreath/outbreath), *muladara/sahasrara* (root/crown chakras), *Shiva/Shakti* (light/power of consciousness) all find balance in the inner stillness supported by effortless steadiness of *asana.*

2.49: tasmin sati śvāsa praśvāsayor gati vicchedaḥ prāṇāyāmaḥ

Asana having been perfected, regulation (vicchedah) of breath by a pause in either inhalation or exhalation constitutes a pranayama.

For Patanjali, a *pranayama* is either an inbreath and a pause, or an outbreath, with a pause. The Sanskrit *vicchedah* means to pause and observe. What do we observe when we are sitting quietly, we exhale, then pause before taking the next breath? We observe that when the breath stops, the mind stops. The mind is inextricably connected to the breath. We observe the natural stillness that occurs with every breath. With this regulation, we have an everpresent reference to the transcendent with each *pranayama.*

To better understand the term *pranayama*, *prana* is the life force of the conscious indweller that enlivens the body. *Ya* means to bring forth, and *ma* is to nurture. Through *pranayama* we bring to consciousness the flow of life itself.

2.50: bāhyā 'bhyantara staṁbhavṛttir deśa kāla saṁkhyābhiḥ paridṛṣṭo dīrgha sūkṣmaḥ

Pranayama has external, internal and stationary operation, and when observed according to space, time and number, becomes long and subtle.

During meditation we can carefully observe the natural unregulated breath patterns over time and we will discover that when we are the most relaxed and centered—physically, mentally and emotionally—the breath is slow and shallow. When we are intensely focused on an object of meditation, or absorbed in the bliss of the Self, we find that breath may naturally become suspended for a period of time. Because of the reciprocal influence of breath and mind the practice of breath regulation emulates these naturally occuring patterns and entrains the mind to its most peaceful repose.

Patanjali refers to external (*bahya*), internal (*abhyantara*) and stationary (*stambha*) operation; meaning outbreath, inbreath and suspension. These terms do not have the same meaning as *rechaka*, *puraka* and *kumbhaka*, as used today. *Bahya* refers to the outbreath followed by the natural pause (*stambha*) at the bottom of the breath. *Rechaka* is the expulsion of the breath; not quite the same as *Bahya*. In the same way *kumbhaka* is the intentional supression of breath; *stambha* is the natural stillpoint between the breaths.

Space, in this sutra is external and internal. External space extends from the tip of the nose to the point where the breath is extended. Internal refers to the space inside one's body. Into the internal space we breathe *prana*: the life energy of the conscious indweller. Our primary intention is to make conscious this influx of *prana* enlivening the body. Visualize the *prana* as it enters the heart center and spreads to the soles of the feet and the crown of the head. Actually feel the scintillation as the *prana* tingles through every nerve channel into every cell. This practice infuses purifying energy through all the *chakras* and awakens dormancy in the higher centers of consciousness.

Time is determined in three ways; none of which is clock time. *Kshana* is a moment in time that it takes for the repetition of a *mantra*. For example; if the *Pranava OM* is used as the *mantra*, one *pranayama* may take three *kshanas*; or may be extended to five *kshanas*. The other unit of time measures one complete *pranayama* (*bahya* plus *stambha*) and is called a *matra*.

Pranayama by the numbers uses a unit of time called *udghata*, which is the extent of time that *stambha* (supression) does not cause uneasiness.

In the framework of Astanga, *pranayama* is practiced to make the breath both long and subtle. Subtlety is attained when a fine cloth held at the tip of the nose does not move. Fineness of *pranayama* in perfected *asana* prepares the mind for attainment of *samadhi*—the objective of Astanga Yoga.

Pranayama as a *Tantric* practice aims to awaken *Kundalini Shakti*; but nowhere does Patanjali mention *Kundalini*.

2.51: bāhyā 'bhyantara viṣayā 'kṣepī caturthaḥ

The Fourth (chaturthah) pranayama is transcendent to external and internal operations.

It is curious that Patanjali calls this transcendent *pranayama* "The Fourth" and not by any other name. Perhaps he is making a reference to the state of consciousness referred to in the Madukya Upanishads as "The Fourth" (the other three being waking, dream, and deep sleep). The Upanishad tells us:

> The Fourth, say the wise, is not subjective experience, nor objective experience, nor experience intermediate between these two, nor is it a nega-

> tive condition which is neither consciousness nor unconsciousness. It is not the knowledge of the senses, nor is it relative knowledge, nor yet inferential knowledge. Beyond the senses, beyond the understanding, beyond all expression, is The Fourth. It is pure unitary consciousness, wherein awareness of the world and of multiplicity is completely obliterated. It is ineffable peace. It is the supreme good. It is One without a second. It is the Self. Know it alone!
>
> (The Upanishads. Prabhavananda & Manchester. Vedanta Press. 1947. P. 75)

We will not be surprised that the state of awareness of the Fourth *pranayama* is the same as that given in the Mandukya Upanishad. The Fourth can be described as a spontaneous period of breath suppression following a practice of progressively long and subtle *pranayamas*. The spontaneous suppression may occur sitting calmly in *asana*. Breathing is diaphragmatic with little movement in the chest. The body feels light with a pleasant sensation from breathing *prana* into the whole body space. *Pranayama* slows and lengthens becoming extended and subtle. The mind becomes quite still, imagining an infinite boundaryless void. The inner sound (*anahata-nada*) may be heard ringing lightly from the movement of the *prana*. In the perfect stillness very little *prana* is required to sustain the body and the breath eases effortlessly into quiescence. This is the transcendent Fourth *pranayama*. Body awareness fades, time stops, there is no thought content, one is only conscious of consciousness itself.

The Fourth is arrived at by long practice of *asana*, meditation and *pranayama*. *Asana* must be steady and comfortable. Meditation must be imperturbable. *Pranayama* must be controlled with the practice of extending *bahya*, *abhyantara* and *stambha* with subtleness. The body must be strong. Diet should be simple and light with a minimum of animal fat. Fasting is a quickener. The Fourth *pranayama* comes in its own time.

2.52: tataḥ kṣīyate prakāśā 'varaṇaṁ

From the Fourth pranayama, the veil over the light of consciousness (prakasha) is lifted.

Prakasha is the light of consciousness by which everything else is known. We spend our life focused upon the contents of awareness. In the contentless void of the Fourth *pranayama*, all we can know is the intelligent knower; all we see is that which is looking. We come to the final discovery of who we are; our fundamental and true Self. The inner light is the light of awareness, the witness of the appearance.

2.53: dhāraṇāsu ca yogyatā manasaḥ

Thus the mind becomes fit for concentration (dharana).

The Sanskrit root of *dharana* is *dri*, meaning "to hold." In general, *dharana* means to hold mental concentration on an object, practice or teaching. Specifically in Astanga *pranayama* it points to the ability to keep inner concentration on emptiness so that no object distracts immersion in the Self—the light of consciousness knowing itself (*prakasha*). In this capability the mind is fit to attain the highest through *asana, pranayama* and meditation.

2.54: sva visayāsaṁprayoge citta svarūpānukāra ive 'ndriyāṇāṁ pratyāhāraḥ

When the mind is withdrawn from sense-objects, the sense-organs also withdraw themselves from their respective objects and thus are said to imitate the mind. This is known as pratyahara.

The senses are slaves to the mind and go wherever the mind directs. If the mind is fascinated with the contents of awareness, the senses reach out into the appearance and bring the mind all the juice the mind has an appetite for. If the mind turns inward, becomes quiet and directs its gaze to the joyous equanimity of just breathing in and breathing out, the senses also become quiet. So we see here that *pratyahara* is the mind withdrawing from external stimulation and focusing on the inner landscape; thus the senses likewise become withdrawn.

As a practical matter we can't always sit crosslegged in the dark breathing in the bliss, but we can remain centered in the inner quiet as we live our life. *Pratyahara* can be cultivated so that the senses are not such a distraction when we are focused on the task at hand.

2.55: tataḥ paramā vaśyate 'ndriyāṇāṁ

As a result of these means, there follows control over the senses.

Asana provides a firm foundation of stillness for the mind to find equipoise. *Pranayama* provides a focus of the mind to draw inward and regulate the flow of *prana. Pratyahara* is the focus of the mind to internal process that thereby constrains the senses from their external sense-objects. Thus the senses are controlled when the mind loses interest in the external and becomes immersed in the internal realm of *prana* and Self-awareness.

This state is first awakened in the firmness of *asana, pranayama* and depth of meditation. It does not stop there, however; this state of Self-absorption can be taken into the world as a state that permeates all activity as we go about our life.

Book 3: Siddhis

3.1: deśabandhaś cittasya dhāraṇā

Dharana is fixing the mind on one object.

The final four practices of Astanga Yoga are inner practices, so *dharana* is best applied to inner objects or qualities; although one may also take an external object for *dharana. Dharana* is an exclusive concentration in that the mind does not wander to other interests or distractions.

Let us take, for example, a *dharana* on evenness of breath in *pranayama.* The body is steady and comfortable in *asana*, the senses are withdrawn and indifferent to their objects, mind is still—*vrittis* restrained; the attention is focused on the quality of evenness in the inbreath and outbreath. We can extend the length and subtlety of the breath keeping evenness with a slight constriction of the pharynx, as in *ujjayi*, but with little or no sound. In *stamba* we pause to rest momentarily in the utter stillness of *asana*, breath, and mind knowing only the witness of the practice. *Dharana* on evenness is continued through the repetition of *pranayama.*

3.2: tatra pratyayai 'katānatā dhyānaṁ

One-pointed steadfastness of the mind is dhyana (meditation).

Like *dharana, dhyana* is steady concentration, but *dhyana* is a continuous focus of attention to an object, quality or state, rather than intermittent. More importantly, in *dhyana* the object is irrelevant; the state of unchanging, undisturbed calm can be applied to any object, quality or action. Becoming established in *dhyana* is the natural result of steady practice of *dharana.*

The state of *dhyana* is no longer concerned with the contents of awareness, but resolves the artificial duality between intelligent consciousness and the objects of perception. The appearance is looked upon by the impartial witness.

3.3: tad evā 'rthhamātra nirbhāsaṁ svarūpa śūnyam iva sāmadhiḥ

In meditation the true nature (svarupa) of the object shines forth, not distorted by the mind. That is samadhi.

In this description of Astanga Yoga we have been given several practices—*asana, pranayama, pratyahara*, etc.—but *samadhi* is not a practice. It is a shift in identity from the ephemeral corporeal self to the conscious indweller. When "that which is looking" sees the appearance, it appears in its true nature (*svarupa*) undistorted by thought, feeling or personal history. The shift to the witnessing Self is persistent; *avidya*, ego, attachment, aversion and fear have burned away in *sadhana.*

Samadhi does not mean withdrawing from the world; it only means that we see clearly that which is, without distortion from the mind. Because of the inner fulfillment in the blissful state we are no longer needy of things from the world—materially, emotionally or spiritually. We are finished with the wheel of *karma* as all our actions are performed without motive. We are happy and content, just being.

3.4: tryam ekatra saṁyamaḥ

The practice of dharana, dhyana and samadhi together is samyama.

It may seem redundant to call these three meditations upon an object by the same name, but in practice, it is not. External or internal objects of contemplation may be complex or subtle and thus may have multiple facets to know in various depths. To fully know an object the meditator may focus simultaneous threads of *dharana, dhyana* and *samadhi* on different faces of the knowable. *Samyama*, thus, refers to the complete process of knowing an object.

3.5: taj jayāt prajñā lokaḥ

By the mastery of samyama, knowledge becomes wisdom.

Mastery is measured in degrees of absorption in an object; and in practice, results in the exclusion of all other objects. This is true of external objects of the world, internal objects of the mind, and the knower itself. This sutra refers to the knowledge of the Self; as *prajna* means supreme knowledge. In this case we apply the concentration of *samyama* to *Purusha*, the Self, to the exclusion of external and internal objects, to become established in the liberated state of *kaivalya*. This begins with *dharana*: glimpses of inner stillness when the mind relents the pestering of *vrittis*. With practice, we meditate deeply (*dhyana*) upon the witness of the mind. Ultimately *samadhi* is our natural state; we become the inner stillness knowing the appearance as it truly is. This is wisdom.

3.6: tasya bhūmiṣu viniyogaḥ

Mastery is attained in stages.

There are three gates on the path of mastery; each one must be passed through in sequence, and none skipped. The first gate is *samyama* on an object of knowledge. Absorption must be complete and exclusive. The second gate is absorption in the senses, free of the mind: knowing the world with no reaction to it. Finally, absorption in awareness knowing itself. This is liberation (*kaivalya*).

3.7: trayaṁ antaraṅgaṁ pūrvebhyaḥ

These three limbs are more internal than the previous five.

Dharana, dhyana and *samadhi* are internal practices, *yama, niyama, asana, pranayama* and *pratyhara* are more external.

3.8: tad api bahiraṅgaṁ nirbījasya

But these three are external to nirbija samadhi—without seed.

As refined as *samyama* is, the focus is upon some knowable. *Nirbija samadhi*, having no object, is awareness absorbed in itself as radiant, self-luminous consciousness whose nature is equinimity and bliss.

3.9: vyutthāna nirodha saṁskārayor abhibhava prādurbhāvau nirodha kṣaṇa cittānvayo nirodha pariṇāmaḥ

Nirodha parinama is the transformation of the mind in which the mind becomes permeated by the condition of nirodha (stillness), which intervenes momentarily between an impression that is disappearing and the impression that is taking its place.

This sutra looks at the mind in the process of changing state from fluctuation to stillness (*nirodha parinama*). The mind has a manifest layer and a latency layer. When information is acquired by the mind, the fluctuation of mentation is stored as a *samskara* in the latency layer. The more this information is accessed or referred to, the stronger the *samskara* becomes making the latency more accessible to the manifest layer. Impressions come and go between the manifest and latency. There is a space of stillness between the impressions, and that, too, creates a *samskara* of mental stillness that likewise exists as latent impression. However, even when the mind is still, the latent impressions are still active but do not come to awareness.

There are two states of the mind: fluctuation and stillness. These states flow back and forth, one being dominant and then the other, depending on the activity and dominance in the latency layer. As the *samskara* of stillness increases, there is an upwelling momentum of stillness in the manifest layer. In this increase, the stillness begins to displace the *samskaras* of active impressions. At a critical point there is a sea change in the mind of stillness dominance. This point is described as *nirodha parinama*.

As this dominance increases further, active *samskaras* are completely displaced. Once that happens fluctuation *samskaras* no longer arise because the dominant stillness is the nature of consciousness itself.

Information continues to be accessed and referred to but active *samskaras* no longer form due to the dominance of stillness.

3.10: tasya praśānta vāhitā saṁskārāt

Steady practice of tranquillity assures a serene mind.

For inner serenity to be sustained, one must be persistent in the state of the impartial witness. This will maintain momentum of the latency of stillness, thus displacing the formation of distracting *samskaras.*

3.11: sarvārthatai 'kāgratayoh kṣyayo 'dayau cittasa samādhi pariṇāmaḥ

Samadhi parinama is the gradual settling of distractions and the simultaneous rising of one-pointedness.

In previous sutras, *nirodha parinama* is shown to bring a peaceful inner state from which the appearance can be surveyed without disturbance. In *samadhi parinama,* attention is focused upon a single object of contemplation, and all other distractions fade from awareness. *Samadhi parinama* also implies that the attention can be sustained over a period of time; be it an external object, an inner subtle object such as *anahata-nada* (the inner sound), or concentration upon unity of the seer where the perceived, perception and the perceiver is unified.

3.12: tataḥ punaḥ śāntoditau tulya pratyayau cittasyai 'kāgratā pariṇāmaḥ

The mind becomes one-pointed when the subsiding and rising thought-waves are similar. This is ekagrata parinama.

One-pointedness is the emphasis of this sutra. *Ekagrata* is a further refinement of *samadhi parinama,* in that, *samadhi* can be a concentration on cognition that arises from latent *samskara.* In *ekagrata,* the single pointed concentration is in the fulcrum of balance between arising and subsiding thought. We can think of this balance point also as a zero point of pressure between the urge of thought and the urge of supression; there is complete equilibrium of movement.

The focus is absolute and no other distractions pull the attention away from *ekagrata parinama* concentration. There is effortless presence in the light of awareness.

3.13: etena bhūte 'ndriyeṣu dharma lakṣaṇā 'vasthā pariṇāmā vyākhyātāḥ

In ekagrata parinama, knowledge of an object goes beyond the sensory, visible, temporal and conditional properties.

Objects are known by their various characteristics. We observe change over time and project change into the future. Objects have density, form, color and utility. Objects can also change state and manifest different attributes. The mind is full of associations by which we appreciate objects. *Samskaras* shower the mind with *vrittis* about the object of observation. Have you noticed?

In *ekagrata parinama*, there is one-pointed focus on its essence, as it is, right now. In this undistracted direct knowing, everything is revealed in all permutations, in all time.

3.14: śānto 'ditā 'vyapadeśya dharmā 'nupātī dharmī

The substratum is inherent in all characteristics in each object in nature whether they be active, latent or unmanifest.

Everything is made from the same substratum (*dharmi*). Given this intrinsic unity, any object can change into anything else in time as the active, latent and unmanifest characteristics mutate. Essentially everything already is everything else, the substratum being preserved. The active characteristic is known in the present, the latent is known in the future and the unmanifest is known in the past. At the deepest level, knowing anything is knowing everything. At a superficial level, whether clay is plant food or a fine vase, it is still clay. Whether gold is a coin or a pendant, it is still gold. Beyond this there is the intrinsic unity of clay and gold, being of common substratum.

If we think we know some object, we may in fact know only the active, but mutable, characteristic and know nothing of its latent or unmanifest characteristics. It is not until we know all characteristics down to its immutability of substratum that we truly know an object. The essential substratum of all *prakriti* is vibrational patterns of energy (*spanda*).

3.15: kramānyatvaṁ pariṇāmānyatve hetuḥ

The variation in transformation is caused by the variety in the underlying process.

The variety of characteristics available to the substratum of nature gives a great variety of objects in various stages of evolution over time. Each characteristic can be a substratum for a further generation of transformation, ad infinitum. The awakened yogi looking out upon the diversity but seeing only the substratum, lives as the impartial witness to the objects in a phenomenal world.

3.16: parināma traya saṁyamād atītā 'nāgata jñānaṁ

Practicing samyama on the three stages of change brings knowledge of past and future.

All things are revealed to the power of perception purified by meditation. The simultaneous practice of *nirodha, samadhi* and *ekagrata parinama* is the process of changing our mental potential from incomplete to total comprehension. This can be applied to external objects or concepts. In this sutra, the power is applied to the characteristics of an object, its change over time and its state (active or inert). By this process one can see its past and future.

The yogi will notice this effect as a matter of course in the practice of *samyama*. There is little use in pursuing this power for entertainment. It is enough to know that it happens.

3.17: śabdā 'rtha pratyayānām itare 'tarā 'dhyāsāt saṁkaras tat pravibhāga saṁyamāt sarva bhūta ruta jñānam

The word, its implied object, and idea behind a word are mixed in the mind in a confused state due to superimposition. By performing samyama on the sound, separation happens and there arises comprehension of the meaning of sounds made by any living being.

Let's look closely at what happens when someone says the word "ocean." You hear the audible syllables, the mind reaches into memory and connects to the strongest ocean *samskara*; you get a mental picture of that memory or fantasy; then you superimpose that image into an estimated context that comes with the original word, "ocean." This happens in a flash, all at once, then the mind rushes off to the next association in the word string.

Often it happens that our cognitive and emotional associations are different than the speaker's and we feel confused when there is misunderstanding.

This sutra says that when we perform *samyama* on the sound, that we will understand. This separates the original word from our inner zoo of *samskaras*. We concentrate intently in stillness to receive the full communication; no matter the language or source.

3.18: saṁskāra sākṣātkaraṇāt pūrva jāti jñānaṁ

By observing past impressions through samyama, knowledge of previous births is obtained.

It is the subtle body that carries impressions of *kleshas* and *karmas* from lifetime to lifetime. We know that in the stillness of meditation we are pelted by all kinds of impressions that arise from memory, from *samskaras* in this incarnation, and *vasanas* from previous lifetimes. By one-pointed concentration upon these impressions we are able to discern knowledge of discrete lifetimes by collecting threads of *karmas* and *vasanas* together.

3.19: pratyayasya para citta jñānaṁ
3.20: Na ca tat sā 'laṁbanaṁ tasyā viṣayī bhūtatvāt

Through samyama the thoughts of another can be known. But perception through samyama does not bring knowledge of the mental factors that support the contents of another's mind.

When our concentrated mind is utterly empty, it is possible to be aware of another's thought. We must, however, be able to discriminate ambient impressions from our own cognition. Even though these external perceptions may be accessable, we can not know the memories and *samskaras* that originate the other's thought processes.

3.21: kāya rūpa saṁyamāt tad grāhya śakti staṁbhe cakṣuḥ prakāśā saṁprayoge 'ntardhānaṁ
3.22: etena śabdā 'dyantardhānam uktaṁ

By performing samyama on the form of the body to suspend receptive power, the contact between the eye of an observer and the light from the body is broken, and the body becomes invisible. Similarly, sound, etc., is suspended.

By the practice of *nirodha parinama, samadhi parinama*, and *ekagrata parinama* upon the subtle energy of the physical body, one can discern the specific function that makes the body visible to others. The power of *samyama* is applied to interrupt the dynamic of perception so that the link between the perceiving eye of others and the visible energy of the yogi is suspended and invisibility occurs. Similarly, sound and other sensory impressions are suspended.

3.23: sopakramaṁ nirupakramaṁ ca karma tat saṁyamād aparānta jñānaṁ ariṣṭebhyo vā

By performing samyama on the two types of karma, fast acting and slow acting, or upon omens and portents; the exact time of death can be predicted.

The *karma* from actions performed yields results immediately if the action is of great intensity; or in the course of time if the action lacks intensity. *Samyama* on the intensity or on the chain of action-reaction gives the knowledge of the time and circumstances of death of the body.

The time of death can also be reckoned through *samyama* on omens and portents. an omen, or portent, is a sign of approaching death. These signs are of three kinds: personal, elemental and divine. An example of a personal sign is no longer hearing anahata-nada (inner sound). An elemental sign might be seeing the wraith of an ancestor. A divine sign might be an experience of the blissful and serene boundarylessness of the beyond.

3.24: maitryādiṣu balāni

By performing samyama on friendliness, or any other attribute, great strength in that quality is obtained.

We remember from sutra 1.33 "*...cultivating friendliness toward the happy, compassion for the unhappy, delight toward the virtuous, and benevolent indifference toward the unrighteous.*" In the present sutra we apply the power of *samyama* on the these virtues. In the utter stillness of *nirodha parinama* we drink deeply of happiness, delight and compassion. In the single pointedness of *samadhi parinama* we infuse these virtues into our being. In the absoluteness of *ekagrata parinama*, no other impressions can arise other than happiness, delight and compassion. Not only are we the embodiment of these virtues, all in our presence can not resist reflecting these qualities in themselves; that is, we have the power to give joy and healing in the midst of suffering without being the doer of anything.

3.25: baleṣu hasti balādīni

By samyama on physical strength one can gain the strength of an elephant. The same is true of other strengths (such as mental, moral, psychic and spiritual).

The example of the elephant is likely symbolic to represent the scale of power that is attainable through the use of *samyama* directed at the ability of our choice—physical, mental, moral, psychic or spiritual.

3.26: pravṛtty āloka nyāsāt sūkṣma vyavahita viprakṛṣṭa jñānaṁ

Through samyama on the intelligent light of consciousness itself, is revealed knowledge of subtle, hidden and distant objects and phenomena.

Essentially, there is nothing anywhere hidden from the inner light of intelligence that is persistently one-pointed. This is not an exploration by the senses, but with the power by which the senses are awake. Nor is this an inquiry by the mind, as direct-knowing transcends logical cognition. It is because the seer (*Purusha*) is not confined to our cranium but is omnipresent and all-knowing.

3.27: bhuvana jñānaṁ sūrye saṁyamāt

By samyama on surya, the universe is known.

Surya, the solar deity, also signifies the inner Self. The inner *Surya* is located at the heart center, the place where *prana* is breathed in, as the center of sentiency. From here, *prana* is radiated into the rest of the body space, as the sun is the life-giver in our local domain of space-time.

In Vedic lore, the *Suryadvara* (path of the sun) leads liberated souls to *Brahmaloka*. Along this journey the souls pass through various *lokas* corresponding to levels of attainment. These *lokas* are inhabitated by *Devas* waiting to incarnate on the physical plane. *Samyama* on the inner *Surya* reveals the universe of *lokas*.

A realized yogi has the power to become discarnate through the process of wilfully supressing the action and feeling of the body. Last of all the sentient portion of the *sushumna* and inner *Surya* can be given up, sending the soul along the path of the sun to *Brahmaloka*; from which there is no return. The crown *chakra* at the opening of the *sushumna* is known as the *Brahmarandhra*, or *nirvana chakra*.

3.28: candre tārā vyūha jñānaṁ

By samyama on the moon comes knowledge of the stars' arrangement.

Knowledge of the stars' arrangement is attained through the kind of sensory acuity of objects that are known by reflected light. Moonlight is but reflected sunlight. Similarly, acuity of the senses is but a reflection of the light of consciousness by which everything is known. Souls bound to the senses leaving the body take the path of the moon through the senses and must return for another incarnation. One who lives by the light of consciousness itself is no longer bound to the senses and leaves the path of the moon for the path of the sun.

3.29: dhruve tad gati jñānaṁ

Through samyama on the pole star comes knowledge of the stars' movements.

If one becomes so still in their focus on the pole star, the movements of the stars will be seen; similarly, movement of inner *prana* is referenced by one's own inner stillness.

3.30: nābhi cacre kāya vyūha jñānaṁ

By samyama on the navel plexus, knowledge of the body's constitution is revealed.

Before technology came of age in medical practice, the best way to know the physical body was through direct knowing. This, of course, is divined through deep meditation upon the organ systems of interest.

3.31: kaṇṭhakūpe kṣut pipāsā nivṛttiḥ

By samyama on the pit of the throat, cessation of hunger and thirst is achieved.

During long meditation, various bodily discomforts arise. *Samyama* can be used to bring ease to the body in a contemplative *asana.* Among these, hunger and thirst can be alleviated through one pointed concentration at the *Vishuddha chakra*—in the notch at the top of the sternum.

3.32: kūrma nāḍyāṁ sthairyaṁ

By samyama on the kurma nadi, motionlessness in the meditative posture is achieved.

Kurma, literally, means tortoise or turtle. Hindu mythology is rich in imagery of the turtle representing strength and steadiness. the *kurma nadi* is a subtle energy channel that runs from the eyes to the navel plexus. The practice is to focus intently in the center of the lungs to steady the breath. When the breath is steady the mind and body will be steady.

Turtles and other reptiles such as the iguana and snake are known to remain motionless for long periods of time. *Samyama* on the *kurma nadi* brings this characteric stillness to the breath, mind and body.

3.33: mūrdha jyotiṣi siddha darśanaṁ

By samyama on the inner light, one has the darshan of a siddha master.

As the student deepens in meditation, he or she may have experiences of inner lights—a red glow, white light, blue pearl, etc. This light may be accompanied by the appearance of *siddha* master, either living or discarnate. Or one may receive the master's teaching on some point of wisdom, an insight, or deeper stillness. It is good to remember however, that the light is not "it." Inner light is an object of awareness; the Self is the witness of the light.

3.34: prātibhād vā sarvaṁ

Siddhis may also be attained through pratibha (intuition, or inner light of wisdom), thus knowledge of everything arises spontaneously.

Everyone has an occasional flash of intuition—direct knowing beyond any rational deduction. As the student of yoga deepens in meditation, the inner light of wisdom flashes more frequently, but we must learn how to discriminate insight from *chittavrittis*. Through persistence in *sadhana* inner stillness will predominate in the inner landscape and the flow of intuition will increase. Gradually the light of *pratibha* becomes a continuous stream and we can shine this light of wisdom upon all matters.

How do we do this? What attitude must prevail for *pratibha* to persist as steady wisdom?

Notice that at any given moment we are listening to the prattle in the mind. Not that there is anything of redeeming value in the mind, but the fact is we are listening; this is something we know how to do already. In the stillness of meditation we turn our awareness to listening beyond the emptiness. By focusing our listening deep into the boundless infinite we open a conscious channel to the light of wisdom. The shift is subtle yet profound. See what your experience is in listening in on the stillness beyond the mind.

We draw inspiration from consciousness itself. The conscious awareness of the small self (*atman*) is not different from universal consciousness (*paramatma*). This is a fundamental teaching of *Vedanta*. And as Nobel Prize winning physicist Erwin Schroedinger remarked: Just as there is only one physical reality, so also there is only one consciousness.

Patanjali has listed numerous *siddhis* attainable by *samyama* upon various tangibles and intangibles leading up to this sutra about *pratibha*. Here he says that all these *siddhis* are attainable through living in the stream of *pratibha*, the inner light of wisdom.

3.35: hṛdaye citta saṁvit

By samyama on the heart center, the knowledge of the mind-stuff is gained.

The mystical heart is considered to be the center of consciousness and the pure I-sense. Deep meditation in the heart center reveals the workings of the mind. We see that consciousness becomes the mind contracted by objects of perception. Further, we discriminate that it is not the mind (*Buddhi*) that is aware, but consciousness itself is the seer.

3.36: sattva puruṣayor atyantā 'samkīrṇayoḥ pratyayā 'viśeṣo bhogaḥ parāthātvāt svārtha saṁyamāt puruṣa jñānaṁ

The intellect (buddhisattva) and the Self (Purusha) are completely different; the intellect existing for the sake of the Self, while the Self exists for its own sake. The cause of experiencing dualities of pleasure and pain is caused by not distinguishing the two. By samyama on the distinction, knowledge of the Self is awakened (Purusha jnanam).

Buddhi exists to present what is seen or experienced to *Purusha*, the seer. But it is *Buddhi*, the intellect, that must discriminate *Purusha* from *Buddhi*. How can *Buddhi* know *Purusha*? *Buddhi* is mutable *Prakriti* and is endowed with the *Gunas* of *sattva, rajas* and *tamas*. *Buddhi* must overcome its own activity and inertness through meditation to become a predominately *sattvic* (*buddhisattva*) object of the seer; and appears as a simulation of *Purusha*. By *samyama* on this simulation, knowledge relating to *Purusha* is acquired. Upon the cessation of *Buddhi*, *Purusha* becomes self-realized.

3.37: tataḥ prātibha śrāvaṇa vedanā, 'darśā 'svāda vārtā jāyante

From this spontaneous enlightenment follows intuitional hearing, touching, seeing, tasting, and smelling.

After the *siddhi* of *pratibha* (direct knowing) is attained through the practice of *nirodha parinama, samadhi parinama*, and *ekagrata parinama*, supernormal sensory powers arise spontaneously, without concentration. They simply arise of their own, unbidden.

3.38: te samādhāv upasargā vyutthāne siddhayaḥ

These superphysical senses are siddhis when the mind is turned outward, but obstacles in the way of nirbija samadhi.

The yogi comes to a fork in the road once the practices bring *siddhis*. To continue on the path of liberation (*kaivalya*) is to release any attachment to display of yogic *siddhis*, as this will be the source of *chittavrittis* incompatible with inner contentment and serenity. On the path of *kaivalya, siddhis* come and go; they are noticed but do not become a distraction.

That being said, Patanjali continues to recount more *siddhis* in the following sutras.

3.39: bandha kāraṇa śaithilyāt pracāra saṁvedāc ca cittasya para 'śarīrā 'veśaḥ

By weakening the bonds of mind and body, and by knowledge of the workings of the mind, consciousness of self and others is revealed.

The bondage of mind and body are strong because of conditioning of identity. Through the power of concentration and knowing "I am not the body," the ties are weakened, loosening the mind from the body. Understanding the flow of vital energy allows an awakened one to guide others in detaching from the body and remembering the Self. In this way, one whose mind is free may enter, or influence another.

3.40: udāna jayāj jala paṅka kaṇṭakādiṣv asaṅga utkrāntiś ca

By mastery over the ascending udana energy current one accomplishes levitation over water, swamps, thorns etc. and can leave the body at will.

Udana is the *prana* that directs the vital currents of the body upward. Concentration on *udana* provides a feeling of lightness. *Udana* also carries impressions from the senses to the brain. Concentration on *Sattva Guna* in the *udana* current can elevate the body above discomfort.

Focus on *udana* in *sushumna nadi* will facilitate leaving the body voluntarily.

3.41: samāna jayāj jvalanaṁ

By mastery over the samana energy current comes radiance to surround the body.

Samana prana is the vital force responsible for digestion, and nourishment of the entire body; it is located between the diaphragm and the navel. Directing the power of consciousness to the *samana* generates an aura of effulgence and radiance.

3.42: śrotrā 'kāśayoḥ saṁbandha saṁyamād divyaṁ śrotraṁ

By samyama on the relationship between Akasha and the ear, supernormal hearing becomes possible.

Akasha (ether) is one of the five fundamental elements *(maha-bhutas)* and arises from the subtle essence (*tanmatra*) of sound; the other elements being air, fire, water, and earth. *Akasha* is considered to be the eternal all-pervasive substratum that provides the ground for all other substances to exist. *Akasha* is only the medium of sound thus is not a thing that has real existence. There is, however a real relationship between the sense of hearing and *Akasha*. *Samyama* upon this *sattvic* relationship awakens a supernatural sense of hearing. This is the power of clairaudience.

3.43: kāyā 'kāśayoḥ saṁbandha saṁyamāl laghu tūla samāpatteś cā 'kāśa gamanaṁ

By samyama on the relationship between the body and akasha, lightness of cotton fiber is attained, and thus traveling through the ether becomes possible.

Akasha, the formless void, has the property of sound; that is, energy wave propagation with no form. Contemplating the body as nothing but an organization of energy waves, being vacant like *Akasha*, is to think of the relationship between the body and *Akasha*. *Samyama* upon the inner sound (*Anahata-nada*) transforms the I-sense to energy of the *Akasha* and enables the lightness of form and to move effortlessly through space.

3.44: bahir akalpitā vṛttir mahā videhā tataḥ prakāśā 'varaṇa kṣayaḥ

Beyond the body is the light of intelligent consciousness that is not cognitive in nature. It is the universal intelligence that transcends the body. Samyama on consciousness itself removes the veil that covers the light of cosmic intelligence.

It is truly great that we have a rational sense to symbolically represent the world for communication, logic and abstraction. That is indeed the fundamental framework that orders knowledge and society. But there is more than the outer appearance and inner knowledge. We make the leap from knowledge to wisdom going deep into the stillness beyond the veil of the mind. There is revealed direct knowing of things as they are, transparent to currents of *vrittis*. In this eternal limitless space we are free of all that has bound us in ignorance in all our incarnations.

Of the many layers of veils, the most opaque is the bondage of identity with the body. Once this darkness is aflame with the light of consciousness, the others, including the mind, fall away readily in time, and freedom ensues.

3.45: sthūla svarūpa sūksmā 'nvayārtha vattva saṁyamād bhūta jayaḥ

Samyama on the essential nature (gross and subtle), interrelatedness and function of the elements; one sees the essence of all elements of nature.

In the depth of meditation we are witness to thought-objects arising and dissolving. Each *vritti* has its distinguishing characteristic and its unique pull on our attention. But we have learned that objects of mind are, in fact, merely a contraction of consciousness itself. Knowing this, we are not distracted from the bliss of the Self, but remain anchored in the impartial witness as thoughts come and go. In exactly the same way, looking out on the appearance we see objects that call to our senses, but we know the intrinsic unity of the common substratum (Sutra 3.14) and are not distracted. Thus we remain immersed in the bliss of just being.

Attaining a state beyond the reach of pleasure and pain the yogi has the power of indifference to the objects that are the cause of attachment, aversion and fear. This is mastery over the objects in nature.

3.46: tato 'ṇimādi prādur bhāvaḥ kāya saṁpat tad dharmā 'nabhighātaś ca

When the elements are mastered one is no longer disturbed by them. From this mastery comes manifestation of the ability to become minute as well as other powers. Mind and body reach perfection and extraordinary powers become possible.

Through mastery over the elements, one can change appearance to become invulnerable to the adversities in nature.

Even though the yogi may attain *siddhis*, he or she does not interfere with the natural process of the universe as it is. Destiny and *karma* play out without interruption.

3.47: rūpa lāvaṇya bala vajrasaṁhananatvāni kāya saṁpat

Beauty, grace, strength and firm durability constitute bodily perfection.

Attainment of the previous *siddhis* naturally manifests in the perfect integration of body, mind, spirit, nature and breath. The yogi becomes transparent to the inner perfection that resides in each of us as our true nature.

3.48: grahaṇa svarūpā 'smitā 'nvayārthavattva saṁyamād indriya jayaḥ

Mastery over the senses is achieved through direct perception of the senses observing their related objects, how such objects are understood, the cognitive relationship with the object, how the object, the senses, the mind and the Seer are interrelated; and what results from such perception.

There are five levels of acuity in which the yogi understands the senses and their functions, thus gaining power over sensory function. The first level is that of the sensory receptivity so that knowledge can be created in the mind. The second is the distinctive features of the senses, such as the eyes, ears, etc. Third is awareness of the active state of attunement of the sense organs to their objects of awareness. Fourth is the quality of sensing; that is, knowability, activity, and latency of the perception. The fifth level is knowing the senses as instruments for pleasure and pain, as a reference for discrimination between *Buddhi* and *Purusha.*

The power attained through this concentration is transcendence of their influence on our mind and perception. We know the sense objects as they are (*svarupa*) with impartiality. Out of this independence arises undistracted direct knowing that goes beyond the limitations of the senses; even beyond spacetime limitations.

3.49: tato manojavitvaṁ vikaraṇabhāvaḥ pradhāna jayaś ca

When the senses are understood in this way, the senses function with the speed of the mind and there is direct sense perception transcending the sense organs and merging into unity with the primary cause.

Earlier sutras have discussed direct knowing, transcending rational or logical process. This sutra extends this *siddhi* to the senses as remote perception of sensory information not local to the body. In this case we go beyond the spacetime limitation into our transcendent, omnicient consciousness. Objects and events can be perceived remotely, forward and backward in time.

In a hologram, the whole is imbedded in each of its parts. Our local consciousness (*Atman*) is not different than universal consciousness (*Brahman*) and is thus holographic in its transcendant presence. This brings to local awareness remote sensory information available to universal consciousness.

3.50: sattva puruṣā 'nyatā khyātimātrasya sarva bhāvā 'dhiṣṭhātṛtvaṁ sarva jñātrtvaṁ ca

One who realizes the distinction between Buddhisattva and Purusha, attains supremacy over all states of being, and becomes omniscient.

The natural course of sadhana will purify the mind of *rajas* (activity) and *tamas* (inertia), leaving only the serenity of *sattva*. It is a very fine discrimination to differentiate the knower of the mind (*Purusha*) from the *sattvic* mind as an object of observation. The pure knower has no "I" sense, while *Buddhisattva* knows that "I have become still." *Purusha* observes *Buddhi* knowing it is still, but has no sense of I-ness when *Buddhi* has dissolved utterly.

Consciousness becomes absorbed in its own Self-awareness rather than contracting to form *Buddhisattva*. When consciousness withdraws its attention from *Buddhisattva*, the mind dissolves and *Purusha* assumes dominion over all states, becoming omniscient.

Omniscience, here, means direct knowing of the true nature (*svarupa*) of all things in the appearance. On a larger scale it implies knowing the true nature of all things in all time.

3.51: tad vairāgyād api dosa bīja kṣaye kaivalyaṁ

By non-attachment to even omniscience, the seed of bondage is destroyed. Then follows kaivalya, liberation.

While there is nothing inherently wrong with manifesting *siddhis*, attachment to their use does not lead to liberation. The power of omniscience may even lead to the realization that *Buddhisattva* is an obstacle to the independence of *Purusha*. Yogic powers arise from the mind, same as the *kleshas*, and must be attenuated to realize enlightenment. Even *vairagya* (non-attachment) is a function of *Buddhi* and is to be finally discarded.

When *Purusha*, the unchanging, stands alone, not related even to *Buddhisattva*, *sadhana* is complete. The Self looks quietly out on the world, established in the unmoving presence of itself.

3.52: sthāny upanimantraṇe saṅga smayā 'karaṇaṁ punar aniṣṭa prasaṇgāt

Any invitation to demonstrate yogic powers, even from one in authority, is best declined. Pride or attachment to siddhis will bring undesirable consequences.

We begin the study and practice of meditation to still the mind and become established in inner peace. Through the long period of *sadhana*, the practices bring attainments, peace and stillness. As long as we are not distracted along this path we become the embodiment of supreme equanimity, living in the joy of just being. Pride or attachment to the *siddhis* are obstacles to finishing this incarnation as a liberated soul (*jivanmukta*).

3.53: kṣaṇa tat kramayoḥ saṁyamād vivekajaṁ jñānaṁ

By samyama on the present moment one can discriminate true knowledge from the false.

Time is not a substantive reality but is only an imaginary concept. We do experience the persistence of the present, however the concept of time arises from sequences of events built up in memory; thus the abstraction of "past" arises. Similarly, imaginary constructs of sequences not yet present gives us the unreal "future."

Whatever exists in the present is real and true; whatever appears in imagination of past and future is neither real nor true. Deep contemplation of the present allows us to discriminate the true from the false, the real from the unreal.

Time is a quasi-linear, arbitrary metric of change; and certainly a convenience in physics, music and engineering; but it is not real—think of it as a shim that makes the math work. You may verify for yourself.... In the inner stillness of meditation, what evidence of time do you notice? You will see that the only suggestion of time is when words arise related to the concept; words being imaginary and not real, e.g., the word water does not quench the thirst, the thought of light does not dispel the darkness.

Mental constructs, such as time, are called *vikalpa*. The challenge in this sutra is to sustain the state of *nirvikalpa samadhi* (thought-free awareness) in the present, so as to live fully in direct knowing of the reality.

3.54: jāti lakṣana desair anyatā 'navacchedāt tulyayos tataḥ pratipattiḥ

With such discriminative knowledge one is able to differentiate between similar things even if they appear identical.

Direct knowing in the present does not rely on rational deduction, linear comparison, or memory of similar experiences, but gives clear knowledge; even discriminating seemingly identical things.

The most profound discrimination (*viveka*) we ever make in our lifetime is between the mind (*Buddhi*) and the Self (*Purusha*). At first we think that it is the mind that is conscious; but then we learn—and verify in our experience—that the mind and the conscious observer of the mind are not the same. It is this conscious witness that is the indwelling Being of our being. Thus the spell of fundamental misidentification is broken. It is only then that we can know the bliss of the Self and attain liberation (*kaivalya*) from ignorance (*avidya*).

3.55: tārakaṁ sarva viṣayaṁ sarvathā viṣayaṁ akramaṁ ce 'ti vivekajaṁ jñānaṁ

This direct knowing is comprehensive and transcendent. It is the pristine truth arising from unconditioned and undivided intelligence in the eternal present.

There are numerous ways the mind gains knowledge: direct perception, inference, *agama* (words of the wise), misunderstanding and imagination. This knowledge is mediated by the mind and is discussed in sutra five of book one. Direct knowing is beyond all these.

Direct knowing arises in the inner stillness when the mind is out of the way. Unbounded consciousness illumines for us whatever we need to know when we need to know it. In the leap from knowledge to wisdom, we first notice, in the occasional flash of intuition. In the silence of meditation we begin to have more and more insight from the nameless formless. Once our inner gaze is continuously directed beyond the inane chatter of the mind and the contents of awareness, we can live immersed in the wisdom of direct knowing. We become the fullness of unbounded consciousness free of mind/body limitations.

3.56: sattva puruṣayoḥ śuddhisāṁye kaivalyaṁ

When the mind (buddhisattva) attains the same purity as the Self (Purusha), there is liberation (kaivalya).

Spiritual *sadhana* is a process of purifying the mind of nescience, ego, attachment, aversion, fear, activity and inertia. Through discipline in meditation the mind gradually relents to contentment in the inner stillness. In that equanimity the bliss of the Self shines through. *Buddhi*, in its purity, reflects only the Self.

We know that consciousness becomes the mind contracted by the objects of perception. Pure *Buddhi* has been purified of objects from *vasanas, samskaras*, memory, imagination or projection; thus consciousness remains uncontracted, free and independent. There is direct correspondence between *Purusha* and *Buddhi. Buddhi* becomes perfectly transparent and *Purusha* sees the world in its pristine nature, uncorrupted by the mind. This is liberation.

Book 4: Kaivalya

4.1: janmau ‘ṣadhi mantra tapaḥ samādhijāḥ siddhayaḥ

Siddhis are gained through birth, specific herbs, mantras, austerities, or samadhi.

It is often said that when we take a new body, we pick up where we left off last time. It is suggested in this sutra that if we had developed *siddhis* in previous incarnations that they will persist into this lifetime. We all know people who have some special ability, and their only explanations is, “Gee; guess I was just born with it.” Perhaps you too have some gift that just comes naturally.

Powers of *mantra* and austerities also can reveal special abilities, but on this path of Yoga, it is the state of *samadhi* that will take us into transcendence.

4.2: jāty antara pariṇamaḥ prakṛtyā ‘pūrāt

Spiritual development proceeds through the flow of natural potentialities.

All beings inherently have all abilities and encompass the highest states. Transformation does not impart new ability, but simply encourages development of natural ability that is already present. Already existing deeper awareness simply flows in to the student.

4.3: nimittaṁ aprayojakaṁ prakṛtīnāṁ varaṇa bhedas tu tataḥ kṣetrikavat

Incidental events are never the catalyst of transformation. They merely act by removing obstacles; as a farmer removes stones from a watercourse to irrigate the land.

The practice of yoga, the study of philosophy, or the inspiration of the teacher, do not impart new ability to the student. The final attainment already exists, and *sadhana* just removes the obstacles to progress on the path.

The radiant bliss of the Self is present fully in the stillness of meditation. The source of intelligence whispers in our ear continuously as direct knowing. The veil of ego, however, covers the luminosity of the Self until the obstacles of nescience, ego, attachment, aversion and fear are gradually removed by conscientious *sadhana* on the path of Yoga and meditation.

4.4: nirmāṇa cittāny asmitā mātrāt

Mind is created from ego-sense alone.

Ego is fundamentally a sense of separation from its source: the pure light of consciousness. When consciousness contracts itself into a separate individual, mind (*Buddhi*) is created, and operates from the illusion that it is different and separate from the knower: *Purusha.* As long as *Buddhi* continues its differentiation outwardly, union (yoga) becomes more and more remote. Only when *Buddhi* turns inward does it reunite with its true Self.

4.5: pravṛtti bhede prayojakaṁ cittaṁ ekam anekeṣāṁ

Although there are numerous, diverse, active minds, they all have one identical nature.

One interpretation can be that all sentient creatures everywhere have different minds of infinite diversity; but within that diversity the foundation of each mind is the same radiance of pure consciousness. Another way of looking at this sutra is that each of us also creates many minds, or personas, to interact with different situations in life. We have many mind-sets, *dharmas*, wear many hats, assume many relationships with people, things and ideals. But still, the same seer (*Purusha*) oversees the many facets of ego that projects our *karma* and *samskaras* into the world.

4.6: tatra dhyānajam anāśayaṁ

Of these diverse minds, only that mind born from meditation is free from residue of karma and samskaras.

One who is not at peace, thinks he or she is the doer, and is reactive to the contents of awareness, is in a cycle of re-creation of *karma* and *samskaras* that has no end. Until... meditation awakens the individual to sweet stillness and equanimity. The bliss of the Self interrupts the destructive cycle and returns the mind to its true nature. Meditation is the path to liberation, and liberation is the end of *karma*.

4.7: karmā 'śukla 'kṛṣṇaṁ yoginas trividham itareṣāṁ

The actions of the yogi are neither pure nor impure; but the actions of others are driven by three forces.

Commonly, actions are 1) reactive to our latent impressions of past experiences, 2) *karma* that is yet unspent, or 3) limitations such as nescience, ego, attachment, aversion and fear. The result of these actions are generally beneficial, harmful, or a mix of the two. This is seemingly unavoidable living in the world. Unless... one has transcended, or become purified of, the cause of reaction. Such a yogi performs whatever action is necessary without burden or drama. Thus there is no karmic action, because there is no doer: no ego-sense of doership.

4.8: tatas tad vipākā 'nugunānāṁ evā 'bhivyaktir vāsanānāṁ

From these karmas, impressions and limitations proceed the development of the tendencies which bring about the fruition of actions.

Yoga philosophy teaches that we enter these bodies bearing the residue of previous incarnations. Siddha masters speak of this with certainty. This residue is carried in the subtle body between lifetimes to manifest again when another physical body is acquired.

There are two kinds of residual essence; *karmasaya* and *vasana*. *Karmasaya* is the latent impression of actions performed in previous incarnations. *Vasana* is memory of feelings associated with action and experience. These *vasanas* are triggered when similar circumstances arise in this lifetime; and we wonder why we have this unfounded feeling in certain situations.

Karmasaya and *vasanas* persist in this life until meditation brings equanimity to the mind, and the active and inert limitations (*kleshas*) are purified to *sattva*. Meditation is the end of *karma* and the end of *vasanas*; we are thus freed from the suffering of transmigration.

4.9: jāti deśa kāla vyavahitānāṁ apy ānantaryaṁ smṛti saṁskārayor ekarūpatvāt

Memory and latent impressions are magnetically linked. This cause and effect link remains even through intervals of time, place or context.

Repeated actions create tendencies. These tendencies imbed deep patterns in memory that persist over time, in different places and in various contexts. These *samskaras* and *vasanas* preprogram our response to future events and circumstances. That is, unless these tendencies are burnt away through meditation. Living in the inner stillness gives no response to the upwelling of tendencies and are thus weakened and eventually dissipated.

In our typical state, latent impressions arise unbidden into our mind. We naturally react to these thoughts and feelings with more thoughts and feelings. *Vasanas* are weakened by returning to the awareness of our physical form in the present moment. This stops the ruminations cold that were chasing each other in our imaginary universe. It's a simple thing to drop out of our imagination back into the body in the present time. The hard part is to remember. Practice.

4.10: tāsāṁ anāditvaṁ cāśiṣo nityatvāt

The desire to live is eternal; thus also the impressions prompting a sense of separate identity are beginningless.

It is just our nature to want to perpetuate our life. Because of this we have lifetimes of impressions related to our dualistic existence; that is, separation from the Self. From this grows the *karmas, vasanas*, and *kleshas* of this separate being. We overcome this separation by returning to the presence of the great Self through the practices of discrimination (*viveka*) and non-attachment (*vairagya*).

4.11: hetu phalā 'śrayā 'laṁbanaiḥ saṁgṛhītatvād eṣāmabhāve tad abhāvaḥ

The tendency to avidya and suffering is held together by cause, effect, basis and support. When this coherency no longer exists, the tendencies vanish.

We know from previous sutras that the cause of suffering is *avidya* (not knowing the Self). This ignorance of our true nature (*svarupa*) gives rise to ego, attachment, aversion and fear. All these imaginary mental *kleshas* dissipate upon knowing the radiant, self-luminous and serene Self. The means to this liberation is not through analysis of the causes. This merely plunges us deeper into the abyss of mental confusion and does nothing to extricate us from the mind. Only the mind suffers. Thus we must make the leap into the knower of the mind from the entanglement of impressions in the mind.

The entantaglements happen in this way: A mind that is prone to restlessness is the progenitor of *vasanas*. When the tendency of fluctuation is destroyed by discrimination and non-attachment, the mind remains as *buddhisattva*, cutting the roots of nescience.

4.12: atītā 'nāgataṁ svarūpato 'sty adhva bhedād dharmāṇāṁ

The past and the future exist in the object itself as form and expression, there being difference in the characteristics.

Whatever object exists has a cause and is knowable. Objects exist in the past, present and future. In the present, knowable objects may exist as tangible form. In the past they exist as memory; and in the future as unmanifest potential form.

Anything caused always exists either as manifest or unmanifest. Unmanifest is not the same as non-existent. Nothing nonexistent can become real, nor can anything real become nonexistent. Even though time (as a concept) is not real, objects are real, even though they may become non-manifest.

This sutra refers to mutable objects, but not the eternal uncaused subject—the silent witness of manifestation. This silent witness sees the manifestation in its true nature (*svarupa*), not limited by past *samskaras*, future expectations, but in the pure reality of the present.

4.13: te vyakta sūkṣmā guṇātmānaḥ

Characteristics of objects, whether subtle or manifest are determined by the nature of the gunas.

It would be useful here to revisit Book 2, Sutras 18 and 19. Patanjali details characteristics of objects as *prakasha* (knowable), *kriya* (active) and *sthiti* (inert) and calls these qualities the *gunas* of *Prakriti*. All objects, both manifest and unmanifest are knowable; that is, they have the *guna* or quality of knowableness. Their manifestation may be active or inert.

4.14: pariṇāmai 'katvād vastu tattvaṁ

The essential quality of any object consists in the uniqueness of proportions of the three gunas.

There is unity in the constantly changing diversity, as all nature (*Prakriti*) is made of the same substratum (*dharmi* [see sutra 3.14]). There is also diversity in the unity provided by various proportions of the *gunas* in each object of *Prakriti*, subtle or manifest.

4.15: vastu sāṁye citta bhedāt tayor vibhaktaḥ panthāḥ

The same object is seen in different ways by different minds.

When an object is perceived, instantaneously, association with *vasana* and *samskara* is made through memory; then arises a story for the context of the object. Everyone will have different associations for each object in the appearance. One must be established in the impartial witness to view the appearance as it is in its true nature, else some spin will obscure the perceived object in its natural context.

4.16: na caika citta tantraṁ vastu tad apramāṇakam tadā kiṁ syāt

The existence of an object is not dependent on the perception of only a single mind.

If we accept that the seer and the seen are separate and not causally related, then an object is knowable by many and its perception is not defined by a single mind. The actual cognition of a knowable varies with the individual, but its knowability is common to all.

The intrinsic nature of a thing is what it is, independent of what different minds may think about it. Furthermore, a knowable exists independently of a mind's perception of it.

You may wonder why it is even necessary to articulate something so obvious, but some scholars think this sutra is a rebuttal to another school of philosophy of the time that asserts that reality is dependent upon the mind.

4.17: tad uparāgā 'pekṣitvāc cittasya vastu jnata jñātaṁ

Things become known or unknown by the way they color the mind.

There is a natural magnetism between the mind and its objects of perception. Whether or not an object is perceived depends on the strength of attraction. If there is a significant affinity, how the object appears to the mind depends upon latent impressions waiting to connect. The strongest *samskaras* related to the perception flood the mind with memory, attitude and expectation. The mind knows only its projections about its perceptions.

Closely examine your own perceptions. Doesn't the coloring (*uparaga*) in the mind give meaning to what you see? Do you feel the magnetism, the hunger for meaning? Doesn't the meaning arise from past experience or future expectations? Perhaps even *vasanas* of other incarnations bind you in interest for no apparent reason.

Only the Self in stillness knows an object as it is.

4.18: sadā jñātāś citta vṛttayas tat prabhoḥ puruṣasyā 'pariṇāmitvāt

The divine unchanging Self is the knower of the changing impressions of the mind.

The outer universe is constantly changing and is reflected in the inner mirror of the mind and its movement of thought. All perception of the inner and outer universes is illumined by the unchanging Seer, pure consciousness. Here, Patanjali points again to the fundamental discrimination between subject and object that is the essential starting place of meditation *sadhana*. Without knowing the knower, the Self is never revealed. Without the predominance of *Purusha* over *Prakriti*, *kaivalya* is never attained.

4.19: na tat svābhāsaṁ dṛśyatvāt

The mind is not self-luminous because it is a knowable object.

Consider the mind as a container; a container of all our thoughts, feelings and memories. As such we can watch the changing mirage in this container. But who is the watcher? It is the self-luminous inner Self. It seems to be our common experience that the mind is the knower and seer, but no; the mind is but the conduit, recorder and commentator of impressions to the Seer. How is it that *Purusha*, the Self, is self-luminous? How can consciousness be aware of its own being? That is it's nature. Consciousness is the light of illumination by which everything else is known and has the power to know itself. This is the fundamental miracle of creation. We verify this in our own experience sitting quietly in thought-free stillness. Looking inward to just being, we know the knower: conscious self-awareness.

4.20: eka samaye co 'bhayā 'navadhāraṇaṁ

Awareness cannot perceive both subject and object simultaneously.

Consciousness becomes the mind contracted by the objects of perception. Consciousness has either the form of objects or the form of the silent witness: the Self. It cannot be both at the same time.

Simply put, the job of the mind (*Buddhi*) is to think thoughts. No thought; no mind. Consciousness can know the mind but the mind cannot know consciousness.

An interesting thing happens when we imagine the mind to be the container of thought, memory and feelings; if we turn our awareness to this **container** of mental content, suddenly the content dissolves, the mind becomes empty. Look at the mind, and it enters stillness. The mind cannot do these two things simultaneously; it is either entangled in thought, or it is quiet (*buddhisattva*) as it emulates the stillness of the Self.

4.21: cittā 'ntara dṛśye buddhi buddher atiprasaṅgaḥ smṛti saṁkaraś ca

We cannot assume that a second mind illuminates our thinking mind, else a confusion of memory occurs.

Presuming that the watcher of the mind is another mind is like infinite regression in a pair of mirrors; and this obviously isn't the case. The mind cannot be the subject and an object, but only an object observed by *Purusha*—pure, self-luminous consciousness.

4.22: citer apratis aṁkramāyās tad ākārā 'pattau sva buddhi saṁvedanaṁ

Self-cognition is realized when consciousness assumes that unchanging form in which there is no movement.

The Unchanging is the conscious being of all that is. The Unchanging is so unchanging that it neither comes into, nor goes out of existence. From the creative power of the Unchanging emerges the mind that creates a diversion for the eye of the Self. This imaginary distraction is the illusion of that which changes. It is, in fact, a passing dream of the Unchanging and is, therefore, not real—a mirage of the ephemeral on the horizon of the Eternal.

We first experience the Unchanging not by its presence but by its absence. Its absence comes to us as the insecurity of being alone. We are like a rudderless boat being buffeted about, without anchor in the storm. The mind seeks everywhere for something to hold on to. Little does it know. We grasp at the ephemeral only to find sand slipping through our fingers. Happiness is a moving target.

In the kaleidoscope of change, seek only the Unchanging. The seeking instinct is inborn to all sentient creatures. We seek outwardly as a matter of reflex. However, the seeking must be turned inward to reveal the Unchanging. Of course, it is at the bottom of the pile of all the wonders there to discover as we turn inward. We can know the Unchanging, not by thinking about it, but by not thinking about it. We touch the Unchanging in the utter stillness of meditation. Here is the safe harbor where we anchor against the winds of change, tides of impressions and storms of feelings.

We become the Unchanging through steadiness of character that reflects the inner stillness we practice in meditation. This is our home, our true nature, our source and goal. Here we find our Self; the end of our seeking and the beginning of perfect contentment.

4.23: draṣṭṛ dṛśyoparaktaṁ cittaṁ sarvārthaṁ

The mind colored by both the seer and the thing seen, knows all.

Buddhi (intellect), purified of activity and inertia, is sentient; thus perceives sensory and mental impressions. *Buddhisattva* presents these experiences to *Purusha*, the seer, as knowable objects of awareness. *Buddhi* knows not only these impressions but knows about *Purusha* through *Samadhi*. The mind can be colored by pure awareness in the same way that it is affected by sensory perception. Thus, when the mind awakens to the Self—as well as its customary sensory and mental impressions—it is all-comprehensive. In this way, the mind presents *Purusha* to itself for its own enlightenment.

Shifting the bias in the mind toward the Self brings liberation from the contraction and superimposition of common awareness. Persistence in this purified state brings absorption in the Self—the state of *Kaivalya*.

4.24: tad asaṁkhyeya vāsanābhiś cittam api parāthaṁ saṁhatya kāritvāt

The mind, though variegated by innumerable tendencies, exists for another in association.

The mind performs numerous sentient functions driven by *vasanas, samskaras* and *kleshas*; but to what end? Is the complexity of the mind for its own benefit?

The mind acts for the benefit of the conscious Self. The mind is not separate from consciousness, but **is** consciousness that has taken the form of physical and subtle knowables. The mind thus acts in concert with—and in the service of—its eternal infinite Self.

4.25: viśeṣa darśina ātmabhāva bhāvanā viniv ṛttiḥ

When one sees the distinction between mind and the Self, confusion ceases about the nature of the Self.

Previous to spiritual awakening we commonly identify with the body, the mind and our personal history. Through *sadhana* and right understanding we see that pure consciousness is the indweller and knower of the mind and body. We have answered the question, "Who am I?" We know our true nature through the sublime state of *samadhi*. There are no further questions for the mind to ask about our identity. The mind merges into that from which it has emerged.

4.26: tadā vivekanimnaṁ kaivalya prāgbhāraṁ cittaṁ

Then the mind—inclined toward discriminative knowledge—gravitates toward the state of liberation.

The inclination toward discriminative knowledge likely began many lifetimes ago; turning inward overcoming outer-directed tendencies, acquiring much new learning and diligent practice of austerities. Persistence of this little-traveled path has brought us here to a steady progression toward the state of liberation.

There comes a point where more thinking about it only keeps us from it, and knowing about it is not it. We must only be aware of just being. In this state of awareness a marvelous thing happens. We typically divide our awareness into two domains: the outer (objects in the appearance) and inner (thoughts, feelings and personal history). Absorbed in the Knower, the mind and its contents shifts to the outer domain of appearance; then there is just impartial awareness enjoying the play against the background of stillness from which the play arises.

4.27: tacchidreṣu pratyayā 'ntarāṇi saṁskārebhyaḥ

Distractions may arise from past impressions, interrupting the practice of discriminative knowledge.

When we first experience the bliss of the Self through *viveka* and *vairagya*, the mind does not suddenly want to be quiet. *Vasanas* and *samskaras* persist, but through *sadhana* the latent impressions are gradually thinned until inner stillness predominates.

Losing interest in our ego, attachments, aversions and fears weakens the power of *samskaras* to interrupt the bliss of the Self. This occurs over time, with persistence. Once the mind is purified, even the practice of discriminative knowledge is released, leaving only perpetual *Kaivalya.*

4.28: hānam eṣāṁ kleśavad uktaṁ

These distractions can be removed as in the kleshas explained before.

In Book II, Patanjali gives the practices that can be used to overcome the obstacles to attaining full consciousness of the inner Self: In 2.1 is prescribed self-discipline, study and recitation of sacred texts, and absorption in the true inner Self. In 2.10 practicing the state of the silent witness thins out the *kleshas* until they subside into dormancy. In 2.11 it is asserted that through meditation the fundamental discrimination between the mind and the Self is made. Sutra 2.26 says that we become established in the identity of *Purusha* through the persistent practice of *viveka*—discriminative knowledge.

4.29: prasaṁkhyāne 'py akusīdasaya sarvathā viveka khyāter dharma meghaḥ samādhiḥ

Disinterest even in the highest knowledge, and immersion in Self-awareness, brings a state of samadhi like a rain of virtue.

In our life of *sadhana*, we strive for attainments of the most sublime knowledge and experience. In the end, we will release even the most noble desires and rest in the silent state of just being. This state of utter freedom is called *dharmamegha-samadhi* and is characterized as a cloud of *dharma*. Living in a desireless *dharma* where there is nothing to gain or lose, the body does what needs to be done without burden or drama. The mind is without impulse and no *karma* is created. The indweller rests in immutable serene contentment.

4.30: tataḥ kleśa karma nivṛttiḥ

From this there follows freedom from karma and kleshas.

In the state of *dharmamegha-samadhi*, the obstacles of nescience, ego, attachment, aversion and fear have been burned away in *sadhana*. The mind has dissipated and *karma* destroyed. One becomes *jivan mukta*—liberated while still in the body. When the indweller departs the body there is no affinity that calls out for the causal body to return from the supracausal. One is finished on the plane of suffering.

4.31: tadā sarvā 'varaṇa malāpetasya jñānasyā 'nantyāj jñeyam alpaṁ

Then all the veils and impurities of infinite conscious intelligence are totally removed. Whatever remains to be known is insignificant.

Impurities referred to here are *gunas* and *malas*. There are three *malas* that bind the individual soul to transmigration: *anava-mala, karma-mala* and *mayiya-mala*. *Anava mala* is the first forgetfulness. When we awaken to the world, we forget that we are the divine presence of pure consciousness. *Anava* is the root mala and is the last bond to be dissolved. *Mayiya mala* is the sense of differentiation. We experience this in the thought that I am this body and my Self is different from another self. *Karma mala* empowers the empirical person to create *karma* due to actions performed under the bondage of *mayiya mala.*

Buddhisattva, the *guna* of unlimited knowledge, is the power within *ekagrata-samadhi* to fully realize a knowable. However, this power is attenuated by the coverings of *rajas* and *tamas*—the *gunas* of restlessness and inertia. Through *dharmamegha-samadhi, rajas* and *tamas* are dispersed and unbidden power of direct knowing arises.

Once the veils and impurities fall away, common knowables hold little interest, being conditioned and finite. The light of freedom (*kaivalya*) reigns supreme.

4.32: tataḥ kṛtārthānāṁ pariṇāma krama samāptir guṇānāṁ.

Then the gunas terminate their sequence of transformations because they have fulfilled their purpose.

All *Prakriti* is subject to the natural causal law of the *gunas.* Being causal, there are effects that naturally occur in this realm of the changing. The empirical self is associated with the beginningless changing until the unchanging Self—*Purusha*—presides in the place of the empirical self. When the self becomes the Unchanging *(dharmamega-samadhi)* the purpose of the *gunas* is finished and the causal laws cease to function in relation to the Self.

Practically speaking, when the yogi attains liberation, the *rajasic* and *tamasic* tendencies of the mind come into balance with *buddhisattva.* In the stillness of balance there is no further sequence of cause and effect. The mind goes into latency, leaving conscious awareness knowing only itself in the eternal present.

4.33: kṣaṇa pratiyogī pariṇāmā 'parānta nirgrāhyaḥ kramaḥ

The sequence referred to previously is an uninterrupted succession of moments. Change is recognized at the end of the sequence.

A principle is eternal when its essence is not destroyed even during change. The *Gunas* are constantly in changing balance but the *Guna* principle is the eternal nature of *Prakriti. Purusha* also is eternal but is changeless. *Gunas* change through a sequence of momentary and incremental change, thus a sense, or concept, of time sequence arises. In immutable *Purusha* there is not the sequence of moments; only the eternal present. Thus for one who is mentally focused on mutable *Prakriti,* time exists moment to moment. For the yogi established in the eternal present of *Purusha* there is no sequence of moments and no cause and effect. We remember the Zen story of the crow that lands on a branch, the branch breaks and the crow flies away. In the Zen mind the crow does not cause the branch to break because there is no cause and effect and everything happens in the present with no sequential relationship to imaginary past or future.

Once established in the eternal unchanging *Purusha,* the false notion of time comes to an end.

4.34: puruṣārtha śunyānāṁ gunānāṁ prati prasavaḥ kaivalyaṁ svarūpa pratiṣṭhā vā citiśakter iti

The characteristics of the mind, having no further purpose, resorb back into its true nature of pure consciousness. Thus consciousness alone exists, free of contraction, immersed in itself.

We know that consciousness becomes the mind, contracted by objects of the appearance. *Buddhi* serves *Purusha* as a conduit of sensory information. But the impartial witness, not hungry for sensory entertainment, is content within itself. *Buddhi* fades away from lack of interest and merges back into that which gave it form.

Kaivalya means absolute transcendent oneness, liberated from matter and transmigration. The finished yogi does what needs to be done, without motive; radiant in the tenderness of selfless love.

Index

T

V

Y

Made in the USA
Middletown, DE
09 September 2024

60498357R10080